The Savvy Patient

The Savvy Patient

How to Be an Active Participant in Your Medical Care

David R. Stutz, M.D.
Bernard Feder, Ph.D.

and the Editors of
Consumer Reports Books

Consumers Union
Yonkers, New York

Library of Congress Cataloging-in-Publication Data
Stutz, David R.
    The savvy patient : how to be an active participant in your medical care /
David R. Stutz, Bernard Feder, and the editors of Consumer Reports
Books.
        p. cm.
    Includes bibliographical references.
    ISBN 0-89043-313-5
    1. Medical care—Quality control.   2. Physician and patient.
    3. Consumer education.   I. Feder, Bernard.   II. Consumer Reports
Books.   III. Title.
R727.S78   1990   89-77116
610.69′6—dc20   CIP

Design by The Sarabande Press
This book is printed on recycled paper ♲
Third impression, May 1993
Manufactured in the United States of America

The sample hospital consent form on page 129 courtesy of Sarasota Memorial
Hospital, Sarasota, Fla. The "Durable Power of Attorney for Health Care" form
on page 240 reprinted by permission of the American Association of Retired
Persons (AARP), Washington, D.C. The "Florida Declaration" on page 235 is
taken from the Florida Life Prolonging Procedures Act, *Florida Statutes* 84-58, ss.
765.01–.15 (1984), courtesy of Concern for Dying, New York, N.Y.

Contents

Acknowledgments

We want first to acknowledge the contributions of the many patients whose concerns and questions inspired this book and suggested its format.

Thanks are due Herbert Hall, our agent Bert Holtje, and our editor Tom Blum, whose interest in and enthusiasm for the project helped us to transform it from a proposal into a plan. We owe a debt of gratitude to the medical librarians at Sarasota Memorial Hospital, Sarasota, Florida; New York University Medical Center; and Cabrini Medical Center, New York, for their expert assistance in locating the materials that fleshed out the plan.

Finally, we owe special thanks to our wives, Karen and Elaine, for their support and encouragement, for their patience, and for the constructive criticism they offered through multiple drafts and numerous revisions.

The Savvy Patient

Introduction

You wouldn't be likely to relinquish control over your life savings to a stockbroker who had been recommended to you by a friend. Yet most people unhesitatingly entrust their bodies and their lives to doctors about whom they know almost nothing and will permit these doctors to make decisions for them about everything from ingesting powerful drugs to undergoing major surgery. In no other profession that involves relationships between free adults is the authority and the decision-making power vested so heavily on one side.

Historically, physicians have taken for granted that they owe their patients only their skills and their best judgment, certainly not the obligation to share decision-making. The rationale for this strange accretion of unilateral authority is the notion that the physician, as a result of his or her specialized training, knows what is best for the patient. However, in today's world, with the explosion of sophisticated treatment options, each with its unique mixture of benefits and risks, and each with its expert champions, it is becoming more and more difficult to assume the existence of a common interest between the patient and any individual doctor. Your medical treatment is far more likely to be determined by the particular biases of your attending physician or by the field in which your doctor specialized than by informed choice or even by the "informed consent" that has become a buzzword in medical circles. Instead of the process of mutual decision-making that is suggested by the phrase, the doctrine has come to stand for the legitimization by the patient of the doctor's unilateral professional decision.

Such unilateral power is corrosive. Not only does it corrupt the doctor-patient relationship, but it warps the judgment of doctors themselves by denying them the feedback that is essential in rational decision-making. The remarkable power granted to physicians in our society has led some to assume the mantle of authority as evidence of their superior, if not infallible, judgment. Others, painfully aware of their fallibility, their shortcomings, their uncertainties and self-doubts, hide behind their authority as a shield against questioning from outside the profession. For within the profession of medicine, despite the procedural safeguards that are designed to ensure accountability, professional solidarity and an elaborate code of professional etiquette tend to protect even the grossly incompetent from exposure. This isolation from criticism promotes another sin that is at least as deadly as hubris: as self-acknowledged stewards of the public interest in health, doctors have found it difficult to avoid confusing this interest with their professional and personal self-interest.

The kind of medical authority that is exercised today in the United States is of fairly recent vintage, with roots in a combination of events. The most significant of these was the monopoly granted during the middle of the nineteenth century to one of several rival groups of physicians and healers. The victors were those who practiced the kind of medicine that is considered both "traditional" and orthodox medicine today; its adherents believed that the most practical way of combating disease was to rely on drugs and surgery. The losers were homeopathic practitioners and naturopaths.

Militant and exclusive, the orthodox practitioners established a growing network of medical schools. In time, their numerical superiority over rival groups and their increased public visibility and clinical success brought them the political strength to gain control over the admission and training of physicians. This they achieved through licensing laws that barred from the practice of medicine those who advocated other forms of treatment. To this day, the relationship between organized medicine and government is paradoxical and uneasy. On the one hand, licensed physicians depend on government to support and enforce their exclusive control over medical practice. On the other hand, they tend to resist vigorously as unwarranted intrusion all other efforts to regulate the profession.

An irony of the political triumph was that it really wasn't necessary in order to confirm the winners' claim to preeminence in medical practice. It came on the eve of a revolution in medical research that was spearheaded by physicians who were searching for more effective medicines, and it was consolidated at a time when medical science was on the brink of making spectacular advances in the treatment of infectious diseases and of medical and surgical emergencies. But the jealousies engendered in the struggle to protect the prerogatives of physicians intensified an attitude that persists to this day: the notion that the gulf between physicians and their patients is too great to permit shared decision-making.

The claim to medical authority based on the scientific superiority of orthodox medicine itself rested on the peculiar assumption that because medical research is based on clearly scientific principles, the individual medical practitioner is a scientist. In fact, few clinicians are scientists. By and large, while physicians rely heavily on the newer technologies of diagnosis, most practicing doctors are not particularly well versed in scientific methodology, and many don't thoroughly understand the nature or the limitations of the new technologies. They have learned scientific facts and principles in medical school mainly through lecture, pronouncement, and demonstration, and they apply these deductively in practice. The result is that, in essence, the patient who relies entirely on his or her doctor's judgment is engaging in an act of faith—either in the objectivity and precision of science or in the depth of experience and judgment of the doctor.

It isn't our purpose here to question either the competence or the integrity of physicians. We have only to compare longevity tables with those of the past to recognize that our society has benefited enormously from the combination of increasing knowledge of nutrition and of the environmental influences on health, the remarkable developments in pharmacological research, and the great improvements that have taken place in medical and surgical methods and procedures.

Nevertheless, the allocation of decision-making authority that we have come to accept in the doctor-patient relationship is both unrealistic and harmful. The very advances that have helped physicians in their practices also have pushed them into narrow specializations and limited interests, so that we can no longer assume that a doctor's concerns for a patient are necessarily the same as the patient's own concerns.

Virtually every medical question is only in part a technical one; it is also a question that involves personal and social values. How much testing is enough? Of alternative treatments that are available, which is preferable for you? How much medication should be taken to gain what amount of relief from a problem? At what point do the adverse effects of a course of treatment outweigh its potential benefits?

Moreover, the most important questions aren't really technical at all. These involve the values that are rooted in our personal, religious, and social philosophies. When does life begin? When is life over? How should limited medical resources be allocated? At what point is the promise of an extended life span too costly to consider in terms of suffering and mutilation? Many physicians themselves are becoming increasingly uncomfortable with the scope of the decision-making authority that society has bestowed upon them in an age when our technical capabilities make such decisions so vital.

Obviously, the opinions and advice of experts should be sought and considered, and their treatment skills should be used when appropriate. We don't build skyscrapers without engaging architects and engineers. But neither should we expect architects or engineers to make the fundamental decision about whether we build a skyscraper at all. To the degree that a society permits physicians to make unilateral decisions in the most sensitive areas of social policy and of personal values, such a society has relegated its responsibility to a priestly class. Much of the current "malpractice crisis" can be attributed to a combination of doctor-patient failures in communication, mismatches in expectation, and the phenomenon of unilateral decision-making.

Yet bounded and limited as it has been by the courts, and resisted as it still is by large segments of the medical community, the principle of shared responsibility for medical decisions is a doctrine whose time is at hand. Social pressures codified by legal statutes are facilitating the emergence of dialogue to replace pontification, of information and advice to replace "doctor's orders." Given prevailing medical attitudes and practices, it is not yet reasonable or realistic to expect that doctors will initiate such dialogue. After all, it's not the doctor's interest but the patient's welfare that is best served by opening up the process, though every responsible practitioner eventually will find such a relationship gratifying, we believe.

Sharing decision-making doesn't imply that you are expected to become an expert about the substance of medical practice. It does mean that you must learn more about the dynamics of medical practice and about how medical decisions are made. You must learn what questions to ask and how and when to ask them so you can actively explore the options available to you and make the decisions that you need to make, some even before you enter into negotiations with physicians.

Sharing responsibility for your health care means that you will come to accept in reality the responsibility for decisions that the law assumes you already have when you sign the consent forms that are sometimes thrust upon you in times of medical crisis. When you are truly informed, negotiating over the specifics of your medical care should not only help you achieve your goals without straining the relationship between you and your doctor but should actually strengthen that relationship.

That's what this book is about.

1

The Limits of Certainty

In recent generations, the search for unambiguous answers to questions about physical health has shifted from religious faith to faith in the promise of science. The perception of medical practice today is that it is fundamentally a scientific process in which highly trained professionals can utilize a remarkable array of scientific tools to arrive at precise and certain solutions to medical problems.

With these rising expectations has come a corresponding reduction in the tolerance for uncertainty and ambiguity. People are impatient with questions and demand answers. They assume that if medicine cannot provide the answers they hope for, the fault must lie with incompetent or ignorant physicians. Most of the medical quacks who flourish today do so because they promise the comforting assurances that the knowledgeable and responsible physician cannot offer.

CHANGING VIEWS OF SCIENCE

Generally, many of the heightened expectations about medicine are based on a distorted perception of scientific methods and approaches. The notion that reason and science will provide correct answers can be traced to those Greek philosophers of the fifth century B.C. who saw order where others in the ancient world saw themselves at the mercy of dreadful and inscrutable forces they could only hope to appease.

This notion of scientific certainty reached its height with the intellectual and scientific revolutions of the seventeenth and eighteenth centuries, the crowning glory of which was the model of the clockwork universe conceived by Isaac Newton. Newton's great achievement was that he made the whole system comprehensible. The universe was a great machine, complex to be sure, but—like any machine—

susceptible to analysis. For Newton, every effect had a cause, and nothing operated by chance.

The faith of many scientists in the Science of Certainty was shattered in the dawn of the atomic age. A new model of the universe began to emerge from the work of atomic physicists—a universe that can be approximated but never completely understood. When it was discovered that the orbits of electrons could not be predicted with any precision, atomic theorists recognized the role of chance in scientific calculation. Even the notion of objective precision in measurement was modified. The physicist Werner Heisenberg's well-known *Uncertainty Principle* states, in effect, that it is virtually impossible to observe anything with complete objectivity, because the very act of observing an object creates a change in its nature or condition.

The Model of Probabilities

This new model of science, on which much of medical research and testing is based, *does* provide an order. But it isn't the order of Newton's clockwork system, in which precise observation was thought to lead to accurate prediction. The order of certainty was replaced with an order of *probability*. This new order predicts not by working from the immutable laws of nature but by estimating odds, by calculating chances, and by constantly revising expectations.

Scientists today generally prefer not to search for immutable truths, an area some of them think should be left to philosophers and theologians. This doesn't mean that scientists no longer *talk* of truth. It means that when they do, they usually are referring to matters with a high order of probability, to the likelihood that their experiments and observations can be reproduced and corroborated, or to the probability that certain things will happen again because they have happened that way in the past. Particular outcomes don't occur because of some absolute causal determinism but because the order of probability makes it likely that they will happen.

The principle of indeterminism or probability means that there is room for the exception, for chance, for the unexplained, and that when such an exception happens, it need not shatter one's belief in the way the system works. Probability means that it's important to calculate the odds. The order of probability may be so high for certain events that it approaches truth. It may be so high that we are willing to stake our very lives on it—as we do every time we drive across a bridge or use an elevator.

Scientists have come to recognize a new mode of decision-making as well: in order to make reasonable decisions, there isn't an absolute need to know everything in advance. Scientists operate by making tentative decisions based on what they know at the time and by making adjustments and corrections if and when problems develop.

The Limits of Medical Research

As in other areas of scientific inquiry, the process of scientific medical research continues to produce more and more information. Unfortunately, the accumulation of data does not mean that medical practice is likely to become more "scientific"—that is, more *certain* in its answers. While medical research is likely to become more effective or efficient in some ways, it offers little promise that such advances will ever eliminate the physician's uncertainty in either diagnosis or treatment. Writing in *The Internist* of January 1986, Dr. William Campbell Felch, the journal's editor, lists a number of reasons why the findings of medical research may not always be helpful to physicians. Among them:

- *Our scientific database is not absolute or monolithic.* Few research studies are in perfect agreement. A determined investigator, writes Felch, can always find somewhere in the vast "scientific" literature a paper that will support any position he or she wishes to take. It is this phenomenon that has permitted quacks to cite respectable references in seeking to bolster outrageous claims.
- *Scientific information seldom is unequivocal.* It rarely tells us that one way always works or that another never does. Here again, both the researcher and the practitioner must fall back on the calculation of probability, not the computation of certainty.
- *Even incontrovertible information may not be helpful.* Antibiotics are useful in bacterial, not viral, infections but, says Felch, "We clinicians have difficulty making timely decisions in individual cases as to whether infections are viral or bacterial and must decide whether to use antibiotics or not in the face of uncer-

tainty," a dilemma which, he points out, is becoming even greater today because of the emergence of newly identified infectious agents, such as those causing Legionnaires' disease.

• *Published scientific studies tend to be one-dimensional.* Studies may provide odds, but in the absence of other data, they may not provide answers to real problems of decision-making. For example, it is well established that postmenopausal women who take estrogen decrease their one-in-ten chance of developing osteoporosis—a thinning of the bones leading to an increased chance of a fracture. But few of the studies answer the questions that most concern doctors and patients when they discuss the pros and cons of taking estrogen: What are the risks of uterine cancer? What are the chances of cutting that risk by adding other hormones, like progestins? Are the benefits worth the costs?

UNCERTAINTY IN MEDICAL PRACTICE

Medical practitioners, like medical researchers, realize that they will never be able to eliminate the problem of uncertainty either from their calculations or from clinical practice. All responsible practitioners are aware that chance and variability have to be calculated into medical interactions and the decisions that may result.

The uncertainty doesn't stop there. Like electrons in the universe of the atom, doctors and patients alike often behave in ways that are unexpected and unpredictable. The responses of both doctors and patients can be affected by the setting in which their encounter occurs, by their recent experiences—by a myriad of variables, many of which we can't even identify.

Medical practitioners are aware of the difficulty in conducting as simple a measurement as the determination of a patient's blood pressure. "White coat hypertension" is a term that describes a common phenomenon in a doctor's office: a patient's blood pressure shoots up just as the doctor or nurse prepares to take a reading. Blood pressure has an extremely variable nature; it changes constantly during the day, frequently from minute to minute. All kinds of factors affect it: movement, long periods of sitting, anger, anxiety and stress, even the time of day. To many patients, the stress of taking the test will itself cause a spurt in blood pressure readings, and patients who take their own blood pressure measurements regularly report that their home readings tend to be considerably lower than those taken in the doctor's office.

In 1988 the Joint National Committee on the Detection, Evaluation, and Treatment of High Blood Pressure recommended that because of the erratic nature of blood pressure readings under different circumstances, the diagnosis of hypertension should be based only on the "average of two or more readings on two or more occasions."

Perhaps the best-known and most dramatic example of the magic that can be performed by just observing and expecting is the *placebo*, the most explicit demonstration of the self-fulfilling prophecy in healing. When the positive expectation of an observer or a healer is communicated to the patient—or when the patient's own belief in the success of the treatment is strong—the patient's condition is often improved not only by powerful medications, but also by sugar pills, snake oil, incantations, and prayers. In fact, the placebo effect itself can be a safer healing agent than can some of the most sophisticated drugs.

The mechanisms through which expectations are communicated are still not completely understood. It is known that they seem to rest not only on verbal messages, but on voice qualities, silences, pauses, and on the multitude of nonverbal messages that we learn to interpret from our earliest days, a form of communication that has been popularized as "body language." It is also known that such messages may often be unintended, because the doctor who is aware that he is giving a patient a sugar pill is not as likely to invoke the magic of the placebo cure as is the doctor who believes that the sugar pill is actually a potent drug. Clearly, there are factors in medicine that the physician may not be able to control or even to identify; the element of chance, of shifting influences, has to become part of the calculation.

Making Medical Decisions

In the world of medicine the model of indeterminism means that it may be necessary to take risks, if they appear warranted, without knowing either the ultimate truth or even all of the facts. Arthur Elstein, a noted medical educator, has described problem-solving in medicine as "the process of making adequate decisions with inadequate information."

Here is an illustration of what can happen in this kind of decision-making: During a routine exam your doctor tells you, "Your blood pressure has been running $^{160}/_{100}$, but before we rush into treatment, we need to know exactly what the problem is. The work-up will include special tests of your blood and urine, as well as a dye injection for X rays of the kidneys, a process known as IVP, or intravenous pyelogram. If the tests don't show any clear specific problem, the condition is conventionally described as 'essential hypertension,' a way of admitting that the cause is unknown."

"Do you have any basis for suspecting that there might be an underlying reason for my high blood pressure?" you ask.

"No," the doctor responds, "but let's rule out these possibilities before we start a program of drugs without knowing the cause. Some of these possible causes can actually be cured by surgery."

To this doctor, the diagnosis of "essential hypertension" is a cop-out, at least until the tests have ruled out a definitive cause. And his approach appears to be reasonable—unless it is recognized that 90 percent to 95 percent of all cases of hypertension *are* "essential"—that is, they can be attributed to no detectable cause. Given this understanding, you should also be aware that the tests proposed are not only expensive, but they involve a degree of risk. The IVP occasionally triggers serious allergic reactions, and an arteriogram carries with it some risk of clotting. Moreover, for those with hypertension, the high blood pressure *itself* is the major cause of damage to body organs. If this risk can be reduced easily with medication, then there is little, if any, need to find the specific cause of the hypertension, and further radiological testing may carry even greater hazards. The doctor in this case apparently has a low tolerance for uncertainty, one of the characteristics of overly "aggressive" physicians (see below), for whom the need to know overrides the risks and costs of intervention.

In the face of uncertainty, responsible medical calculations are based on the order of probability. The key in this case is to estimate the odds from relevant information about the patient in order to ascertain that the patient isn't in a high-risk subgroup for one of the unusual specific causes of hypertension. For example, if a young woman had recently developed severe hypertension, and if her doctor determined that she was not using birth control pills, the doctor would probably be concerned that she might have renovascular hypertension—high blood pressure caused by a narrowing in the kidney arteries.

The doctor would make such a calculation from the patient's personal and family history, from the physical examination, and from the results of basic screening tests. If this information suggested that there might be a curable underlying cause for the high blood pressure, then further testing would certainly be warranted.

More and more physicians are adopting a "pragmatic" or "probabilistic" approach to decision-making that is based on the understanding that they may never know all the details of a patient's problem. The more they do know, the better—within limits. There is a point of diminishing returns, in terms of costs, risks, emotional stress, and anxiety. Often the passage of time is the best diagnostic test available, as long as no harm is done by delaying either testing or treatment. Sometimes the use of medication in the course of a carefully monitored diagnosis or treatment, referred to as a diagnostic or therapeutic "trial," will prevent the need for extensive testing.

The vital element is close follow-up, with the understanding that both the diagnostic and the treatment programs can be modified as circumstances suggest. Both doctor and patient may agree that it is better to act without all the facts at hand than to chase elusive data—unless there are indications that specific information is needed.

Many physicians have come to appreciate the trade-offs in testing: risks and costs versus anticipated knowledge and benefits. Extensive test programs can be expensive and may often be uncomfortable or, as we've noted, even dangerous. The need to know must be tempered by an appreciation of the costs not only in money, but in risk and discomfort for the patient. A high degree of good medical judgment is based on the ability to know when a patient is likely to be at risk for a certain problem, and then focusing on that problem.

THE PHYSICIAN'S WORLD

Given all the variables, including the completely human ones, physicians respond differently to similar situations. Studies in recent years have shown that, for the most part, these differences have relatively little to do with conviction, morality, or levels of knowledge and competence. Instead, they tend to reflect national, regional, and local practices and habits, and the diverse ways people deal with uncertainty.

National Differences in Medical Practice

Where someone gets sick seems to have at least as much to do with the treatment he or she receives as *how* sick that person is. The style of medical practice varies on a broad scale from one country to another, even among countries in which citizens enjoy comparable levels of health and life expectancies. American medicine generally is noted for its aggressive spirit because it's characteristic of American doctors to want to *do* something. Generally, U.S. doctors order more diagnostic tests, prescribe drugs more frequently, and resort to surgery far more frequently than do their colleagues in Europe. American women are considerably more likely than are European women to undergo radical mastectomies, deliver their babies by cesarean section, and submit to routine hysterectomies. Americans are six times as likely to have coronary bypass surgery as are Britons, and in general they undergo surgery at twice the rate of their British counterparts.

The expectations of American patients are an important factor in this more aggressive approach. Americans tend to regard the body as a machine; they tend to perceive themselves as naturally healthy, and when they are ill, they assume that the problem is something to be located and repaired. This view is in contrast with the European propensity to focus on the body's natural defenses. A European physician is far more likely to prescribe vitamins, hydrotherapy, or visits to a thermal spa than is an American doctor. The American view helps to explain the enthusiasm for annual physical checkups, a practice most responsible medical practitioners elsewhere find superfluous. Underlying this perspective is the reliance on American know-how: "If we can put a man on the moon, surely we should be able to cure cancer."

Regional and Local Differences in Medical Practice

Different regions of the United States often show startling variations in medical practice, even from one local hospital market to another. The research technique of *small-area analysis* has made it clear that many medical decisions are determined more by local practice than by medical consensus.

One such study in Maine, by Dr. John Wennberg, found that women who lived in Lewiston were three and one-half times as likely to undergo hysterectomies as were women living in Rockland. Another study, reported by Drs. Philip Caper and Michael Zubkoff, found that a child living in one Vermont community had an 8 percent chance of undergoing a tonsillectomy, while a child living in another community in the same state had a 70 percent chance of undergoing the operation. These differences exist in virtually every area of medical or surgical intervention. For example, Dr. Wennberg found that the incidence of myocardial infarction, or heart attack, was about the same in the California communities of Palo Alto and north San Diego, but the rate of major cardiovascular surgery was 66 percent higher in north San Diego.

Dr. Mark R. Chassin and his colleagues, who conducted a study for the Rand Corporation in 1986, found that in some regions of the United States, the rate of such costly and traumatic procedures as coronary bypass surgery, breast removal, or total hip replacement was nearly three times as great as it was in other regions. In fact, the researchers found about the same rate of difference in more than half of the 123 procedures they studied. Some of the procedures were performed ten times more often in some areas than they were in others.

These differences may indicate that unnecessary medical care is provided in some regions, that insufficient care is provided in others, or even that illness patterns vary from region to region. Yet Drs. N. P. Roos and L. L. Roos reported in the *American Journal of Public Health* that people who live in high-surgery localities are no sicker than those in low-surgery areas. Incomes are comparable in areas with high rates of surgery and in areas with low rates of surgery, as are insurance coverages. The number of specialists in many high- and low-rate areas studied is virtually the same. Nor can the differences be explained in terms of aggressive versus conservative physicians. In the same area, one operation may be performed at a high rate, while another may be performed at a low rate.

The problem appears to be that physicians are responding to local medical practice; until the development of small-area analysis, no opportunity has existed for physicians to compare their practices with those in other areas. It is small consolation that Dr. Robert H. Brook of the University of California at Los Angeles, who has worked on the Rand survey, observes that "there is a huge gray area in medicine where you can do a procedure, and it is going to do neither much harm nor much good. Perhaps 40 percent of medicine falls into this area."

Aggressive and Conservative Approaches

Even within particular geographical areas, physicians can be roughly categorized as either *aggressive* or *conservative*. Aggressive doctors are those who customarily intervene as early and as vigorously as they can. They will order batteries of tests to gather information that might be useful (see chapter 6); they will attempt to track down every abnormality; they are likely to recommend surgery or other corrective and therapeutic measures. They are driven by two needs: the need to *know* and the need to *do* something.

Conservative doctors, on the other hand, prefer to wait. They have a greater tolerance for uncertainty than do their aggressive colleagues. Generally, their approach is based on the recognition that many problems and conditions will resolve themselves with the passage of time, either by disappearing altogether or by becoming clearer and more identifiable. If intervention is required, conservative doctors usually recommend simple procedures first. They are likely to be more concerned than are aggressive doctors with the negative aspects of testing and with the risks of vigorous intervention.

The two approaches can be illustrated by the hypothetical case of a 48-year-old woman with a fibroid tumor—a benign muscular growth—on the wall of her uterus. If she visits an aggressive doctor, she is likely to be advised to have a hysterectomy. The surgery will remove the uterus, she will be told; then the bleeding she has been having will stop immediately, and there will be no further problem. The same woman, visiting a conservative doctor, is likely to be advised against surgery. The operation, which carries the risks that accompany any major surgery, will also expose her to an increased risk of bladder infection or intestinal injury, she would be told. Besides, the physician would point out, fibroids often shrink after menopause; the bleeding may be controlled in the meantime with progesterone.

Keep in mind that, although doctors have characteristic approaches to diagnosis and treatment, they can't always be pigeonholed as aggressive or conservative. An aggressive doctor may be very cautious in some situations, and a conservative doctor may be quick to act and even impulsive under some circumstances.

It is reasonable to assume that you can balance the particular bias of your doctor by asking for a second opinion. You should know, though, that when doctors in either group need consultative help, they tend to turn to specialists who think the same way they do. And because patients often ask their physicians for the names of consultants to corroborate opinions, the so-called second opinion is sometimes far less objective than you might think. (See chapter 7 for a discussion of consultations and second opinions.)

MAKING A MEDICAL DIAGNOSIS: YOUR CONTRIBUTION

Let's suppose that you wake up with a scratchy throat, you're sniffling a bit, and you're sneezing from time to time. If this were hay-fever season, you might suspect that you have an allergic reaction, but it's midwinter. You don't have fever, so it's probably just a cold, you decide, and you make a mental note to drop by the drugstore on your way to work to pick up some cold tablets.

In effect, you have developed a hypothesis on the basis of several symptoms and a few related facts. While your doctor may have more information on which to base his or her decisions, the process by which medical decisions are made is not very different. To be sure, in medical school, students learning the process of diagnosis are cautioned to complete an examination of the patient and to gather all the pertinent facts before they formulate a hypothesis. However, the evidence seems to indicate that doctors don't do this in actual practice.

The divergence between what is taught in medical schools and what is practiced by physicians is illustrated by the findings of the Medical Inquiry Project, a five-year program of research in medical problem-solving carried out at Michigan State University. This pioneering program rigorously investigated and described the thought and problem-solving processes of physicians, including seasoned and respected clinicians. The project's major findings described how physicians actually solved medical problems when they were faced with incomplete information.

Physicians generate hypotheses early. One of the study's most surprising findings was that *none* of the doctors waited until they had all the facts before making their hypotheses. And 35 percent of the physicians made their first diagnostic hypothesis after only 30 seconds of talking with the patient.

Physicians consider a limited number of hypotheses at one time. After making an early hypothesis, the doctor's time is spent either confirming or ruling out the hypothesis.

As a result of these behaviors and processes, several problems can easily occur. The researchers found that the doctors resisted giving up an early diagnostic hypothesis even in the face of new data and that they sometimes tried to fit the new evidence into the diagnostic slots that had already been developed. Furthermore, the doctors sometimes assigned an exaggerated importance to some facts so they could justify keeping an existing hypothesis that did not explain other findings.

Among the conclusions the researchers drew from their observations were:

Physicians often oversimplify issues. We humans have a natural tendency to perceive complex issues in simple form, and this tendency sometimes causes some physicians to disregard information that does not support their hypotheses.

Diagnostic competence is not necessarily a general skill. Expertise in one area of medicine does not guarantee expertise in another. In fact, the diagnostic accuracy and clinical skills of medical students and experienced physicians alike seem to be related to specific problems. It might be more appropriate to think of medical skills in terms of *profiles of competence*, in which a physician is seen as effective in dealing with certain types of problems in particular situations. This is why it is so important for physicians to recognize when they are outside their areas of competence.

·   ·   ·

Precisely because so many doctors tend to make snap judgments, *how* you as a patient present your symptoms and your concerns is an important issue. Remember that physicians tend to diagnose very early in the visit, and then to stay with this early diagnosis even in the face of information that may not be supportive or that may even be contradictory. To allow for this, try to be as clear and direct as possible when you describe your symptoms and your concerns, taking time to establish in advance the order of the agenda for your office visit (see chapter 4). If you suspect that you are being misunderstood, be persistent at the risk of repeating yourself.

THE VALUE OF OPENING
YOUR PERSPECTIVE

Like medical researchers and medical practitioners, patients must consider the role of sheer chance as they deal with the uncertainty that is part of medical decision-making.

The scientist and the clinician must reconcile the knowable and the unfathomable, the certain and the capricious, in some pattern that makes sense. Patients, too, must make decisions that take into account the known and the unknown, matters that can be controlled and matters that defy control. And, like the physician, they must create a coherent system for reconciling these elements with their own perceptions and understanding.

Such a reconciliation can provide you with a useful perspective in understanding the causes of an illness and in predicting the consequences of selecting one course of treatment over another. It can help in ascertaining which, if any, treatment is likely to make a difference, and in establishing as much control over the course of subsequent events as is possible.

This reconciliation can begin with recognizing the two major fallacies in the ways most of us react to illness: the nagging suspicion that something we have done or left undone has created the problem, and the despair that we are entirely powerless to affect what happens next.

THE FALLACIES OF GUILT AND FATALISM

If you engage in guilt-laden thinking, a common and natural response to becoming ill, you may assume that you are solely responsible for the fact of your illness and for your prognosis. This kind of thinking has been enjoying a vogue in recent years: it is frequently assumed that victims of cancer, heart attacks, strokes, and even accidents have somehow invited their problems, either by their personalities or their behavior.

In the extreme version of this approach, *everything* that happens to you is your responsibility. If you hadn't worked so hard, you wouldn't have had that heart attack; if you had eaten more sensibly, you would have avoided that stroke; and if you had worked on changing your personality, you would have avoided cancer. We believe that to accuse patients of bringing on their own illnesses is not only needlessly cruel, but also implies that it is patients who are wholly responsible for whether or not they recover—a burden so great that it often complicates recovery instead of facilitating it.

At the other extreme from guilt is the model of fatalism, which decrees the denial of all responsibility. In this view, everything that happens to us is a matter of luck, of malevolent forces in the cosmos, or of other such mystical powers beyond our control. Like the guilt response, fatalism is a common emotional reaction when we are faced with an apparently overwhelming crisis like injury or illness. As with the guilt response, fatalism is maladjustive because it can immobilize us. Dr. Harold Bursztajn and his colleagues place such reactions within what they label *the mechanistic paradigm.*

They use this term to refer to the assumptions and principles underlying the Newtonian clockwork system: the notion that all events are the result of specific causes, the belief that the relationship between cause and result is systematic and uniform, and the idea that once we have identified the cause, we can always predict the consequences with some accuracy. A corollary is that the cause can surely be determined, and that if the physician knows his business, he or she will not only identify the cause, but see clearly the therapeutic direction to recovery.

Heredity Is Not Destiny

Both responses—guilt, or the assumption that we are responsible for our illnesses, and fatalism, or the assumption that we have no control at all over our fates—rest on a misunderstanding of the nature of probability.

Of course our behavior makes a difference. If we smoke cigarettes, we're far more likely to experience lung cancer or a heart attack than if we don't smoke. But some people who don't smoke develop lung cancer, while some heavy smokers live to a ripe old age without problems. Clearly, even when we do all the right things or all the wrong things, chance plays a role in the effects our behavior has on health. Personal behavior does make a difference. So do our genes. So does sheer chance. The specifics rest on an interplay between behavior and potential, between our genetic inheritance and the things we do— and the imponderable, incalculable, unpredictable element of chance.

Bursztajn and his colleagues emphasize that in order for people to properly use the knowledge of probabilities, two things must take place: First, they must distinguish between those circumstances that are influenced by their behavior and those over which they have no control. Second, in those areas in which the outcomes are determined by chance, they must understand the odds and use their knowledge to guide their decisions. Any analysis of risk factors in any illness or condition must take into account both categories of risk.

The roles of behavior and chance emerge clearly in an examination of the approximately 1.3 million heart attacks that occur each year in the United States, nearly half of which result in death, either immediately or within a year. Heart attacks are caused by combinations of factors, some of which are beyond our control, many of which are not.

Heredity and metabolic predisposition to a high cholesterol level are powerful risk factors, and they vary from person to person. Male gender and age are additional predisposing traits that are outside our individual control. But diet, smoking, blood pressure control, stress, and lack of exercise are specific potent contributing factors that are very much under individual control. Furthermore, evidence shows that if our daily conduct is strict enough to reduce the controllable risk factors, risk can be decreased to a level that is close to normal.

By applying the probabilistic model, someone who is in a high-risk population can view the controllable risks as a challenge that can be met and the uncontrollable ones as an early warning signal to alert him or her to seek prompt attention.

The Importance of Being in Control

An interesting sidelight to some practical benefits of operating within the framework of the probabilistic model emerges from a study by Israeli psychologist Dan Bar-On reported in the journal *Human Relations*. Puzzled by the observation that heart attack patients seem to know more about how fully they'll recover than their physicians do, Bar-On interviewed 89 first-time heart attack patients and their physicians. He asked why the heart attack had occurred and what would aid the patients in coping with it. Physicians and patients often gave different reasons regarding what had precipitated the attack and offered different prescriptions for recovery. In explaining why these attacks had occurred, physicians tended to focus on purely physiological factors, such as obesity and smoking; patients tended to attribute their attacks to troubling circumstances in their lives, such as marriage and work-related difficulties.

More striking than these differences in perception between doctors and patients were differences among patients that seemed to affect their recuperation. The greatest recovery was made by those patients who believed that the attack had been caused by a combination of controllable and uncontrollable factors. These patients, recognizing the contributing role of their own anger and stress, planned behavioral changes as an aid to their recovery. Those who claimed they would be least likely to return to work and to their normal activities were those who thought that their problems were the result of "fate." Those in the latter group, for example, believed that their heart attacks had occurred because they were "unlucky" and that they would recover if they were "lucky."

The probabilistic model seems to offer a practical benefit. The very act of involvement is therapeutic. It gives you, as a decision-maker, a sense of control over your destiny. Especially when you're sick, this sense of control is essential, and even by itself can help you to cope with what has been called "the second illness": the panic that grips you when you're seriously ill.

What You Can Do

Recognizing the role of both behavior and chance is a major step in taking control of your health care. To assess your given risks—those over which you have no control—it's important to discuss with your doctor the implications of your family history and your personal medical history. Identify the other risk factors that are beyond your control: your genetic inheritance, your age and sex, and your occupation.

Once you are aware of increased risks in particular diseases, you can begin to do something to improve the odds against you. Ask your doctor what specific steps you can take to minimize or even eliminate each risk factor. Remember, such risk factors are merely dispositions and tendencies, not predictions, but you should still ask about the warning signs of problems that may result from them. It's also best to ask about the next step: what to do if the warning signs occur.

SUMMING IT ALL UP

Scientists in general have come to accept a model of science in which absolute certainty is a myth. Instead of scientific truths, they have come to settle on scientific probabilities. An important facet of medical decision-making is the consideration not only of the possibility that something will happen, but of the odds that it will happen.

On the basis of this recognition, physicians have come to a new model of decision-making, in which they are more prone to make decisions on the basis of reasonable evidence than on all the evidence it's possible to amass. They distinguish between the *ability to know* and the *need to know*.

The new model of science has also brought into the calculations of probabilities the element of sheer chance. In medicine, this means that doctors and patients alike must distinguish between medical risk factors that are under their control and those that are not. The former suggest a program for behavior change to alter the odds, while the latter sometimes can provide an early warning system. Reconciling the elements of the knowable with the elements of chance provides the best possible perspective for regarding your medical problems and participating in their treatment.

While there are general patterns of medical decision-making, many of the decisions that your doctor makes about your medical care have little to do with medical necessity. There are significant differences in medical practice that are shaped by such factors as your doctor's personality, his or her personal toleration for uncertainty, and the geographical location in which he or she practices.

Studies have identified the general process of medical decision-making and the potential rigidities in your doctor's thinking that may affect your care. The measures you can take to protect yourself against such rigidities include presenting your symptoms clearly, in the order of their importance and as early in the visit as possible.

Neither guilt nor fatalism is a productive response to illness. It is therapeutic to have some sense of control over your problems, for such an attitude and approach may help you recover more quickly than someone who believes that fate controls both illness and recovery.

2

The Concept of Normality

How normal are you? It's impossible to answer this question without comparing yourself with something—a fixed standard, other people, or an ideal—and each comparison may provide a different answer to the question. In addition, the word "normal" itself has several possible meanings. Your understanding of the concept of "normality" may not be the same as that of someone else, and you yourself may use the word to mean different things at different times. If you and your doctor use different standards to measure normality or do not even agree on the meaning of the term, you may very well have trouble understanding each other.

MEASUREMENT AND EVALUATION

One of the reasons there's so much room for ambiguity in applying standards is that people often confuse two very different concepts: *measurement* and *evaluation*. When something is measured, it is simply being compared against an arbitrary scale or standard—an inch, a pound, a second, or a degree of temperature. The measurement alone tells nothing about whether the quantity being measured is good or bad, healthy or unhealthy, desirable or undesirable. When a doctor tells you that your blood pressure is $^{150}/_{95}$, or that your cholesterol level is 230, you're likely to ask, "Is that normal?" What you probably mean is, "Is that good or bad?" You are really asking for an *evaluation* of a specific measurement. The process of converting a measurement into an evaluation depends on a set of standards that's considerably less fixed than the one used for measurement.

For purposes of medical evaluation, there are three ways of looking at information about "normality" as it relates to medical conditions. Consider these three hypothetical conversations between doctors and patients.

Patient One

"I've been getting short of breath when I exercise," the young man complains. "I huff and puff after I run a mile. I've been running over four miles every morning, and I've never been short of breath like this. It isn't normal for me."

"Let me examine you and see what I can find," says the doctor.

As this example shows, your condition or functional performance can be measured against your previous condition or performance to ascertain the degree to which it has changed.

Patient Two

"When I get up in the morning," the 72-year-old woman complains, "my back is terribly stiff and achy. It takes a good half hour before I can really move around."

The doctor nods. "That's really quite normal for a woman your age."

"Are you trying to tell me that it's normal to be in pain?" she asks with some irritation.

This interchange demonstrates the way in which you can be compared with others, most likely for evaluation against a norm or average. However, the average will vary with the populations that are used to establish the norm.

Patient Three

"Your cholesterol level is 230," the doctor reports to a 47-year-old high school teacher.

"What's normal?" she asks.

"Actually, about half the people of your age in this country have levels in this range. But a normal level should be below 200."

Here we note that you can be evaluated against a scale of condition or of behavior that is considered desirable or good. For example, if experts conclude, on the basis of experimental studies, that a particular level of blood pressure or cholesterol marks the division between "healthy" and "potentially dangerous," then this is the standard against which your blood pressure or cholesterol measurement will be evaluated. As research provides additional information, these standards of "healthy" condition or status may change.

The word "normal" is defined in the dictionary as "usual," "regular," "typical," or "natural." It is also used to connote "healthy" or "desirable." For example, it may be "normal" for a smoker to cough, but it's hardly healthy. For the most part, a doctor is likely to use as his or her basis for evaluation the concept of normality as "average"— either for you or for the population group to which you belong.

IN SEARCH OF THE NORMAL PATIENT

The concept of normality has its roots in the statistics of probabilities—the calculation of odds. The first formulation of a theory of probabilities was developed by a 17th-century French mathematician, Blaise Pascal. According to legend, in order to help a patron who was losing at the gaming tables, Pascal developed a full-fledged theory of probabilities, complete with rules and formulas for calculating odds in various situations, and charts and tables for dealing with the distributions of chance. Pascal and his fellow thinkers realized that the theory of probability had applications far beyond those of the gaming tables, and the mathematics of chance has become a valuable tool in many of the sciences.

The statistics that concern physicians and patients are those that describe and predict human characteristics. The principles of probability that apply here are the same as those that govern the calculations in public opinion surveys, in elections, and even in gambling. In all of these situations, the usefulness of diagnoses, predictions, and decisions rests largely on the accuracy achieved in determining the base of what is "normal"—that is, what is usual, regular, typical, or natural.

The study of human statistics is based on a paradox: all humans are alike, and every human being is different from every other human. No two of the billions of humans who have lived on the face of the earth, who live on it now, or who will occupy it in the future, are exactly the same. Each person represents a combination of genes and experiences that have never been put together in precisely those particular proportions.

Even identical twins do not have the same fingerprints or dental structures or personalities. Not only individual features, but movement and gesture patterns, signatures and voices, personalities and habits, tastes and preferences, and biochemical composition render each individual unique.

Nevertheless, all of the differences and variations create a kind of blend from which generalizations can be drawn. The range of height or weight among the members of any race or nationality is far greater than the differences in the *average* height or weight between different races or nationalities. Averages focus on similarities rather than differences.

It is easy to imagine a representative "average" person who will incorporate typical human biological characteristics. Generally, it is this hypothetical person whom your doctor has in mind when he or she first meets you. The problem is that there isn't just one hypothetical average human whom your doctor treats; there are several.

Physicians use the word "average" all the time. They talk of average life spans, average blood pressure, average medical test readings. Sometimes they use the term "normal" in much the same way. What many doctors, and probably most patients, don't realize is that both "average" and "normal" can mean several different things, each with its own cluster of assumptions and implications.

SOME MEANINGS OF "AVERAGE"

Doctors speak of averages when they discuss prognosis—that is, what to expect from a particular illness and treatment. When you are dealing with estimations of survival regarding serious diseases like cancer, it is important to understand just what the doctor is talking about.

Measures Doctors Use

A hypothetical example of seven people with liver cancer shows several ways to look at "average" survival. These people died between 2 and 96 months after their cancer was diagnosed, with individual lengths of survival shown in the table.

AVERAGE SURVIVAL FOR SEVEN VICTIMS OF LIVER CANCER

Subject	Months Survived	
A	2	
B	3	
C	7	
D	8	midpoint = 8 months *median* survival
E	10	
F	15	
G	96	
7 subjects	141 months total	"average" = 20.14 months (arithmetic *mean*)

The *median* is the figure that describes the life span of the person in the middle of the group ranking. Half the people who had liver cancer lived less than eight months from the time they were diagnosed, half lived more than eight months.

The arithmetic *mean* is the form of "average" with which most people are familiar. When people speak of "average," they're usually referring to this calculation. In order to calculate the *mean* survival time for these victims of liver cancer, one adds up the total number of months that all of these people survived and divides by the number of people. The mean survival for this group was 20.14 months.

The major problem with the arithmetic or numerical mean is that an unusual situation can distort the average. For example, if a few people were to live much longer than most of the others, the arithmetic mean would be unrealistically high. In this case, the mean survival is more than twice the number of months of the median, because the figure is distorted by the single long survivor.

One way of getting around this possible distortion is to speak of one-year survivals, five-year survivals, or some similar measurement. Such a figure indicates the percentage of people alive (or, in some studies, disease-free) after a period of time following a diagnosis or after a particular treatment. Survival rates say nothing about average life spans but deal instead with the likelihood of being alive for a certain period of time after a given reference point. This figure yields a more realistic comparison of life span after various treatments than does either the median or the arithmetic mean.

The various meanings of "average" can lead to trouble, because the term "average" can be interpreted in several ways. The odds for misunderstanding grow even greater when the word "normal" is used, so it is important for you to clarify what you and your doctor mean when you are talking about "average" and "normal."

WHAT'S NORMAL ABOUT YOU

Virtually all medical researchers, and most physicians, refer to normality as "usual," "typical," or "expected." Two factors, however, may make it difficult to get a fix on normality.

The first is that, while normality is a concept that rests on a statistical description of the real world, everyone has created a unique mental model of what is normal or typical, based on his or her personal experiences. People compare every new experience and every new acquaintance with their personal models of "normal" to decide if these new experiences or acquaintances are either typical or out of the ordinary in any way. As someone becomes more familiar with a person, the observer's notion of what is normal or typical shifts to what is normal *for that person.*

Because the experiences of people aren't identical, notions of what is normal are not likely to match precisely. As your doctor gets to know you better as a patient, he or she should think of you more as an individual than as a hypothetical human. The question can then begin to change from *What is normal for most people?* to *What is normal for you?*

The second factor that confuses thinking about normality is that the measure of normality varies from group to group. In medical practice, this variation becomes important for people whose chance of having a problem depends on whether they are in *high-risk* or *low-risk* groups. Factors for categorizing people according to risk may include age, race, family histories, personal behavior patterns, occupation, and travel, to mention only a few.

For example, the presence of dark facial hair may be "normal" in some women from the Mediterranean regions, but for the daughter of two fair-skinned Scandinavian parents, the same phenomenon may be an indication of an endocrinologic disorder. Similarly, a physician who examines two 40-year-old men who complain of chest pains will categorize them in terms of risk factors. The patient whose father and two brothers died of heart attacks before they reached the age of fifty is far more likely to have a heart problem than is the patient who has no family history of heart trouble.

The accuracy of diagnosis and of calculating medical odds and chances rests principally on the reliability of identifying the population to which an individual belongs and in determining how commonly the condition occurs in that group. The frequency with which such a condition occurs *in that group or population* is called the *base rate*, or background odds, for that group. The doctor's estimations of base rates can significantly affect the medical treatment he or she recommends. (See chapter 3 and chapter 6.)

Normal According to Whom?

It's quite apparent that the word "normal" is intimately related to the concept of average. In fact, "normal" and "average" are often used as synonyms in the world of medicine. But in many areas of medicine, the term "normal" has come to mean "healthy" or "well."

For the most part we assume that it is *usual* to be free of disease, but this assumption isn't always warranted. In large portions of the American population, "normal" or average levels of weight or cholesterol are *not* normal in the sense of being desirable or healthy. For example, in this country, the average or "normal" blood cholesterol level is 211 for men and 215 for women. Since it is generally accepted that the dividing line between *low risk* and *borderline risk* for heart problems is 200, a "normal" American should be classified as *borderline risk*.

Generally, there is no great problem in taking the view of normal as typical, as healthy, or as typically healthy, as long as we understand how the term is being used in our discussions.

Your Doctor's Normal World

Everyone has his or her own sense of what is normal in the everyday world, and this sense of what is normal and what is expected to happen on any day and in any particular situation is based heavily on personal experiences. Simply put, people remember what they experience, and they think that what they remember is likely to occur in the future. But personal estimates of probabilities can be grossly distorted by particular experiences, especially if those personal experiences are not generally shared by others.

These issues are important in medical practice because physicians remember what they see, and they make recommendations based on what they remember. Clearly, it's important to have an idea of the kind of patients your doctor normally sees. Doctors' practices and their normal worlds vary according to their specialties and medical interests, the age of their patients, and even the habits and practices of the people they see.

People who visit specialists before problems are well defined may undergo extensive testing for diagnostic possibilities that are unlikely, simply because such diagnoses are common among the other patients in that doctor's special world.

If you're experiencing chronic fatigue and you visit a cardiologist, who deals mainly with heart patients, you'll probably undergo an echocardiogram (a sonar image of the heart) or a stress test to rule out heart disease. If you see a pulmonary specialist, most of whose patients have lung problems, you'll probably be given breathing function tests to rule out a respiratory disorder. If you make an appointment with a doctor who focuses on metabolic diseases, you are likely to undergo hormonal analysis, and if you see a rheumatologist, or arthritis specialist, you'll probably have a battery of tests to search for an autoimmune disorder, in which the body reacts against its own tissues. And all of these for the same symptom of chronic fatigue.

While an inappropriate hypothesis formulated by a doctor may delay the appropriate testing, there is a much more serious consideration. If the doctor's usual caseload does not include your particular problem—even though that problem may be neither rare nor unusual—he or she may never even consider the actual cause of your symptoms.

THE RHYTHMS OF NORMALITY

In order to provide the best possible care, doctors need to look beyond the hypothetical average patient to get to know you as an individual. However, not only are you different from anybody else on earth, you aren't the same person at different times of the day and on different days of the month. The better you and your doctor are able to recognize the variations, the better you can both distinguish between the "normal" you and the abnormal, or "sick," you.

Energy levels, moods and behaviors, levels of task efficiency, and thinking patterns are all related to the fluctuations of the body's chemistry and physiology. Virtually every human process exhibits cyclical variations, and these rhythms and cycles can be as short as seconds and minutes or as long as days, months, or even years.

Short-term cycles include the one-second periods of electrical activity in the heart, the four-second gastric and breathing cycles, and the 90-minute bursts of brain activity that occur while you are awake or asleep.

Among the most important of these body rhythms are the daily rhythms that are called *circadian*, a term coined by Franz Halberg of the University of Minnesota from the Latin *circa dies*, or, "about a day." Circadian fluctuations occur in body temperature, digestive function, circulatory efficiency, alertness and reaction times, sleeping and waking, and in the production of all of the hormones like cortisone and thyroid that govern the body's metabolism.

Some processes are tuned to rhythms that are longer in duration than a day. Such cycles may be monthly, seasonal, annual, or even longer. For reasons we still don't understand completely, some of these longer rhythms seem to be more closely correlated with the lunar than the solar calendar. For example, the menstrual period is closer to the 29.5-day synodic lunar month (from full moon to full moon) than to the 30.4-day solar (calendar) month or to the 28-day cycle that is often assumed to be a lunar month and that is frequently cited as the menstrual cycle. Moreover, the average period of human gestation lies closer to the 266 days of nine synodic lunar months than to the 274 days of nine calendar months.

There is considerable evidence that the vast majority of these rhythms are innate and automatic, but they can be modified to a large extent by the environment and by personal behavior. Influences from the outside world that affect the body's rhythms may be natural occurrences, such as the length of sunlight and darkness. Often, however, it is man-made or self-induced factors that play the greatest role in altering daily body variation. The kinds of meals we eat and when they are eaten; the use of substances like alcohol and caffeine, prescription or over-the-counter drugs; work and social stimulation or pressure; and even physical exercise can markedly affect the body's short-term and circadian fluctuation. But some daily activities are repeated so regularly that they themselves become part of the body's daily rhythm.

Although less apparent, longer-term rhythms also affect the body. The seasons affect moods and body physiology. It has long been observed, for example, that peptic ulcer disease is more common in the spring and fall, at times of seasonal change. Psychiatrists are also recognizing the mood changes that occur naturally in the winter, the so-called seasonal affective disorders that may be induced by the shortening of the daylight hours. After all, most other animals display seasonal behavioral responses as dramatic as hibernation, and although human beings may be able to override and suppress pre-programmed behaviors, they are likely to have at least some impact on our lives.

Recognizing the normal variations from hour to hour, day to day, and even season to season is important, because this is the background against which illness occurs. When your physician examines you or treats you, it's necessary to be able to distinguish between the changes caused by normal internal rhythms and routine daily behavior, and the signs and symptoms caused by a new or unusual activity or by an illness.

The Rhythms of Your Body Temperature and Metabolism

A closer examination of the circadian rhythms of body temperature and metabolism is instructive in order to identify the "normal" you and to understand how disease and medications may alter this normal state.

The body temperature is closely correlated with most of the internal circadian rhythms, and it is the best single indicator of the general level of efficiency. Human body temperature is less variable than almost any other human measurement, staying within a range of about one-half to three-quarters of a degree of the 98.6° F norm throughout the day for most healthy people. The oscillations of the temperature cycle and the biochemical cycles that are associated with it are quite predictable, although they may vary somewhat from individual to individual.

During the night, body temperature will drop until about five A.M., when it will start to rise, and about an hour before that, increased quantities of hormones are secreted to prepare for the day ahead. At about the same time, in the majority of people, involuntary muscular activity of the intestinal system will increase. These movements, known as peristalsis, normally prepare the body for the bowel movement that occurs typically shortly after eating in the morning.

Body temperature continues to climb until about midday or late afternoon, although it will peak at different times for different people. The temperature of "morning people," who start the day full of energy, tends to peak before noon and then drop slowly. "Evening people," on the other hand, start slowly, and in general their body temperature response parallels their general level of function and efficiency. The body's production and secretion of hormones like cortisone, insulin, epinephrine, growth hormone, and thyroid also vary in circadian fashion and affect various metabolic functions accordingly.

Implications for Testing and Diagnosis

Knowledge of the body's temperature and metabolism has important implications in both the diagnosis and the treatment of medical problems. As we have seen, one of the standards for medical evaluation is to compare your condition or your performance with your normal condition or performance to find the degree to which it has changed. Because the body is constantly in a state of change, doctors must take some precautions to avoid confusing a real change in your condition with a natural and predictable cyclical change.

Virtually every test that is administered will provide information about a person *at the time of day* and under the specific conditions in which the test was administered, and any observation must be placed in the context of what is normal under those circumstances. Blood pressure tends to be highest in the evening, and in the late afternoon or early evening, the systolic pressure—the upper number—may be as much as forty points higher than the day's low reading, which occurs during sleep. The diastolic blood pressure—the lower number—does not peak until several hours later, around midnight.

In addition, because physiologic measures fluctuate during a 24-

hour period, the results of laboratory tests can fluctuate according to the time that the samples are gathered or the readings are taken.

Such fluctuations may be very important clinically, especially when treatment decisions are based on the test results or observations. For example, an infection caused by an abscess is likely to be accompanied by a body temperature that is perfectly normal in the morning and becomes elevated only in the afternoon. If the doctor doesn't take into account the time of day that the temperature is taken, he or she might stop medications too soon, and the infection could flare.

In women, the menstrual cycle also affects the body's temperature, because after ovulation occurs, approximately in midcycle, the body temperature rises about 1° F, resulting in a "normal" temperature of 99.5° F. This measurement may suggest a diagnosis of infection if this natural variation is not taken into account. On the other hand, this particular natural variation is useful in assessing fertility by helping to determine when a woman is ovulating and is able to conceive.

It should be apparent that because the body follows circadian and other rhythms, repeated observations that reveal a pattern are often much more informative than are isolated tests and measurements. Bear in mind that you change more over several hours during any day than you do from one day to another at the same time of day. You are much more different between morning and night than you are from one morning to the next.

While the rhythms of internal cycles are reasonably predictable, the influence of changing external factors may not be so easily identified or appreciated. Situational stress, physical activity, eating and drinking, and medications must all be entered into the analysis of any test or observation. It is vital to eliminate as much variation as possible so that other changes due to illness or treatment can be correctly discerned.

YOUR BODY TENDS TO BECOME NORMAL

A study conducted at the University of Utah College of Medicine found that although medical doctors and chiropractors use very different methods of treatment, both groups achieved satisfactory results with more than 90 percent of patients who suffered back or neck pain—that is, the pain eventually subsided or disappeared.

Which of the following is the most reasonable conclusion to be drawn from this finding?

(a) That M.D.s and chiropractors probably worked with different patient populations, and each group was effective in its own practice.

(b) That 10 percent of both medical doctors and chiropractors are probably incompetent.

(c) That the recovery from pain for most of the patients had little or nothing to do with the treatment.

In our society, we have learned to seek professional help for many of our pains and discomforts—and for much of our general unhappiness as well—so it may surprise you to learn that (c) is the most reasonable inference from the data. In fact, you may be surprised, too, to learn that the vast majority of all illnesses are self-limiting or self-remitting. Most patients get better by themselves, with or without any kind of outside intervention. Dr. Fletcher McDowell told the participants at a National Institutes of Health conference in 1975 that if the spontaneous recovery figure were much more than about 65 percent to 70 percent, "I suspect there'd be no need for any of us," and that if it were less than 50 percent, "we'd either all be out of work or in jail, I'm not sure which."

This tendency of self-healing is closely connected to a principle that is well-known to statisticians. It is referred to as *regression to the mean*. What this means is that all more-or-less random events tend to cluster around an average; any extraordinary occurrence is likely to be followed by one that is closer to the average or the norm.

A very tall parent is likely to have children who are taller than average, but not as tall as the parent, and very short parents will probably have children who are somewhat taller than the parents are. Very brilliant parents are frequently disappointed in the achievements of their children, and the children of star professional athletes rarely equal or surpass their parents in the same field.

While many of our characteristics are transmitted genetically, the principle of regression to the mean makes it unlikely that humanity will veer significantly from the middle, either in intelligence or physical characteristics, except over an extremely large number of generations. This is why you don't see one-foot-tall humans, even though short people tend to marry each other, or 20-foot-tall humans, though very tall people also tend to marry each other.

The human body is certainly not a conglomerate of random elements, but the body, too, regresses to the mean. A host of mechanisms function to prevent the body and the mind from straying too far off center. Everyone has days of feeling lethargic, dull, perhaps somewhat depressed. Such moods normally don't last long. What's more, when people do snap back, they're just as likely to cross the mean to a state of well-being, or even euphoria. The mood swings of normal people don't usually interfere with their everyday functioning.

As we noted, body temperature and hormonal balances are constantly in a state of oscillation. This dynamic is often referred to as *homeostasis*, a self-correcting process that controls the work of the various organs and glands to compensate for changes in the environment or aberrations within the body itself. However, from time to time, the homeostatic mechanisms that are designed to keep people normal go awry, resulting in a nonfunctional or even destructive bodily response.

Allergies, for example, are caused by the malfunctioning of one of our bodies' natural defense systems—the development of antibodies to fight off foreign substances. Similarly, the glandular production of thyroid hormone, insulin, male or female hormone, cortisone, or other hormones—all part of the orchestration of body metabolism—can be either too high or too low. This breakdown in the body's usually well regulated hormone production can occur because of a failure or an autonomous overproduction of the gland itself, or because of either too much or too little production of the substances that stimulate the gland.

All of this shows that normality isn't a state of equilibrium but rather a process of constant adjustment, a continual striving for balance. The result is that body functions—and mental functions as well—are constantly oscillating around the settings of an individual's personal normality. This drive toward the mean is often cited as the body's remarkable power to heal itself. Voltaire remarked, "The efficient physician is the man who successfully amuses his patients while nature effects a cure."

People frequently misinterpret the manifestations of this statistical principle of regression to the mean. If a patient happens to be in treatment at the time a spontaneous remission—or spontaneous healing—occurs, he or she is likely to credit the physician with the cure. Moreover, many physicians are just as likely to assume that the medicine or the method of treatment was responsible, often reinforcing a misplaced faith in a procedure that is questionable or even useless.

When Should You Call the Doctor?

Even though the body tends to regress to the mean of normality and can heal itself, doctors still play an important role in maintaining our health. While minor illnesses or injuries will resolve themselves in most cases, physicians may be able to relieve the symptoms more quickly. Furthermore, it has been observed that while about 70 percent of all illnesses, bruises, colds, pains, and the like resolve themselves, we can't always be sure that our particular condition falls into that category.

The other major reason for consulting a doctor, especially if symptoms are severe or if they persist, is that the signs of many serious illnesses often are very similar to those of minor problems, or even to your own normal variations. Some heart problems can easily be confused with gas pains or indigestion, and early diagnosis of such an illness can prevent later problems or even save your life.

This doesn't mean, necessarily, that every complaint or problem must involve medical tests or treatment. But if you know your own normal cycles and if you observe the character and pattern of your symptoms, you'll be able to distinguish between those problems that are likely to go away spontaneously and those that are signals that it's time to see a doctor.

THE RHYTHMS OF ILLNESS

Old legends tell of the influence of the moon on behavior—the word "lunacy" is rooted in the lunar cycle—and of the periodic recurrence of disease. While most such tales are fanciful and fantastic, they are based on generations of empirical observation. Modern research corroborates that mood cycles and susceptibility to disease are frequently time-related. So, too, is the response to treatment.

Many illnesses and variations in mood seem to be cyclical in nature. One of the most obvious of these mood cycles is the one associated with menstrual periods, when major hormonal changes take place. While the physiological changes and the behavior and mood swings in women are generally recognized—in fact, the more severe manifestations have been dubbed the premenstrual syndrome—it is not as well known that men may have similar mood cycles that are associated with more-or-less monthly changes in testosterone production.

It has been known for some time that heart attacks tend to occur most frequently in the early morning and midevening hours. Asthma attacks are most common at night. As noted, some diseases, such as peptic ulcer of the stomach or duodenum, can follow a longer cycle and are particularly prevalent in the spring and fall. Of course, some illnesses, such as allergies or Lyme disease (a tick-borne infection), are caused by external agents that are themselves subject to seasonal variations. As the external causes vary, the occurrence of the disease will vary.

Researchers have observed that a clear association seems to exist between the seasons and the incidence of depression, mania, and suicide. For a small category of depressed patients, the connection is so clear that their variety of depression has been labeled seasonal affective disorder, or, appropriately, SAD. These patients, who suffer depression during the winter months, seem to respond favorably when they move to, or vacation in, an environment with longer hours of daylight or are treated with high-intensity light therapy.

An increasing number of diseases, both physical and mental, have been found to follow cyclical patterns that are caused either by internal hormonal cycles or environmental time-related triggers. Actually, no part of the body is completely stable or immune to cyclical attacks.

In addition to physical changes, alterations in mood seem to coincide with changes in sleep patterns or in eating and drinking patterns. Apparently, chronobiological changes that occur in one part of the body can affect the whole organism, often in ways that seem to be unrelated to the original problem.

In spite of all that has been learned about the cyclical nature of illnesses and body reactions, many patients and physicians still neglect to take into account these body rhythms in their diagnoses and their treatment procedures. Curt Paul Richter, professor emeritus of psychobiology at Johns Hopkins University Medical School, has observed that in their practices physicians tend to identify complaints and symptoms as isolated phenomena. Usually, the patient doesn't recognize the recurrent nature of many symptoms or connect them with other events that have taken place. And because physicians themselves tend to be unaware of the time-ordered nature of so many problems and disorders, they frequently neglect to ask the appropriate questions that might help identify the connections. Dr. Norman E. Rosenthal and his colleagues at the National Institutes of Mental Health point out that many patients have never been identified as having SAD because a cycle with a one-year rhythm is difficult for both the patient and the physician to perceive. It took 11 years before the seasonal pattern of one of their patient's depression was recognized.

The more aware you are of the degree to which your body rhythms are a part of your normality, the better you'll be able to recognize true abnormalities and to communicate with your doctor about diagnosis and treatment. Whether or not your doctor recognizes patterns in your symptoms or the recurring nature of some of your problems depends in large part on the way you observe and report them. This means that you bear a major responsibility in the recognition of time-ordered problems.

THE RHYTHMS OF TREATMENT

The time of day makes a vital difference in the body's reaction to virtually every contact with the world. One of the most intriguing and least understood aspects of our circadian processes is the varying ways our bodies and minds respond to toxins, medications, and to medical interventions.

These fluctuating sensitivities mean that your body at one time of the day can shrug off a toxic substance that can cause it major problems at another time. For example, the chemical histamine is released by the body's tissues during allergic reactions, and it directly causes many of the symptoms attributed to allergies. Histamine may create only a minor irritation if it is injected at eight in the morning. But the same dose injected at 11 at night might cause a major eruption. Allergic persons seem to show the greatest sensitivity to allergens at nighttime, and this is when the frequency of asthma attacks is highest. There seems to be a relationship between the body's fluctuating sensitivity to allergic triggers and the levels of cortisone, both in the blood and in the urine, because the highest levels occur in the blood in the early morning and in the urine around noon.

Similarly, research has made it clear that medicines have different effects at different times. Diabetes patients are sensitive to insulin at night, when a small amount can produce unpleasant hypoglycemia with sweating, trembling, palpitations, headaches, and even mental aberrations. These side effects are influenced by the body's natural insulin cycle, which is affected both by circadian rhythms and by the times that people eat. Diabetics are best off when the insulin program includes a large dose in the morning to handle the effects of breakfast and lunch, with a smaller dose at suppertime to cope with dinner and the overnight blood sugar production in the liver.

Because every substance affects the body differently, there is no single rule that indicates the proper time to take medicine or to abstain. In general, the body is far more sensitive to foreign substances during the night than it is during the day. Among the exceptions to this generalization are the body's reactions to two common over-the-counter drugs: aspirin and antihistamines. Both are less effective, or at least their effects are shorter-lived, at night than they are during the day. The effect of aspirin taken at seven in the morning will last up to 23 hours, but the same dose taken at seven in the evening will be effective for a shorter period.

Similarly, antihistamines, which block the action of the body chemical histamine, seem to be most effective when taken early in the morning, when the body's sensitivity to histamine is lowest. They also seem to offer the longest protection against allergic reactions when they are taken at this time. However, antihistamines may also cause drowsiness, an inconvenient and even dangerous side effect, especially for those who must drive during the day. One solution is to take a small dose that will provide adequate protection while it minimizes the drowsiness that may accompany a larger dose.

In the treatment of asthma, rheumatoid arthritis, and a number of other chronic diseases, a standard medication is cortisone, which reduces inflammation. The problem with this drug is that the prolonged use of corticosteroids can suppress the body's own cortisone production and can cause the full, puffy face that is the hallmark of cortisone excess. However, if the day's cortisone treatment is given only once, early in the morning, the side effects can be minimized. (See chapter 5 and chapter 7.)

SUMMING IT ALL UP

Normality is a statistical concept that is based on what one can expect because it is usual, likely, or frequent. In medicine, however, the term may be used as an indication of what is desirable — and what is desirable may not always be what is usual. It's important, when you or your doctor use the term, to be sure that you both mean the same thing.

Because what is usual or likely varies from group to group, it's often useful to think of *normalities*, in the plural. Identifying what is normal for someone of your age, sex, race, and life-style is far more meaningful than trying to assess what is normal for humans in general. This concept of base rate, or how often an event or trait occurs in a reference group, is so important that we repeat it often here.

On a short-term basis, normality isn't a constant. Your body's internal rhythms and your daily activities combine to change what is normal for you throughout the day. What is normal for you in the morning may not be at all what is normal at night. It's particularly important for us to take these changes into account when we are concerned with medical diagnosis and treatment.

Fortunately, your body's functions tend toward normality, and this tendency, a manifestation of a statistical principle known as regression to the mean, shows itself in two ways. Your body's functions oscillate around what is normal for you. Your blood pressure, heartbeat, pulse, cholesterol levels — all tend to come back to your average blood pressure, heartbeat, and cholesterol levels. This statistical regression works to keep you relatively stable.

Regression to a state of normality is also evident in the body's power to heal itself, and as a result, the vast majority of illnesses and disorders are self-limiting. Nevertheless, you may require professional assistance to discern whether symptoms and problems really will regress on their own or whether other diagnostic or treatment approaches may be necessary.

Once you have identified various aspects of your own normality, you will be able to be more sensitive to medical problems — abnormalities — when they occur.

3

Considering the Odds

For the patient, virtually every question in medical decision-making involves an assessment of odds and probabilities: What condition do I have? How sure can I be that the diagnosis is accurate? Which treatment option is likely to be most effective? What are the benefits and risks involved? Most of all, what are my chances—of surviving, improving, or stabilizing?

Most people rely on past experience to establish the rough probabilities that guide their decision-making. For the most part, these personal assessments serve them reasonably well, especially if the decisions involved are relatively simple or if they are the kinds of decisions and problems that are encountered frequently. But when people are faced with situations with which they may be unfamiliar, or when they aren't sure of the nature or the ramifications of the choices they have, they are more likely to miscalculate the probabilities. And when their thinking is clouded by their hopes or their fears, they may not even be able to identify their choices clearly. Sometimes when we are faced with particularly complex issues, certain quirks in our thinking seem to distort our perceptions of the alternatives available to us.

All these factors that interfere with rational decision-making—an unfamiliar situation, lack of information, strong impulses of hope or fear—are precisely the ones that are likely to be present when you must make important medical decisions. Fortunately, because such distortions in thinking about choices and odds are predictable, it's possible to take measures to guard against them.

DEFINING THE PROBLEM

The scholars who deal with the methodology of the behavioral sciences sometimes refer to the odds and probabilities that govern a given situation as "the rules of the game." One persistent problem in communication between doctors and patients, or between doctors and doctors, is that they may be playing by different rules—that is, for a variety of reasons, they may perceive the odds differently. More to the point, they may be playing different games without recognizing that fact.

Odds and probabilities in a given situation depend largely on the ways that you and your doctor perceive the problem. If you and the doctor have different problems and different goals in mind, you may have trouble dealing with what appear to be simple decisions based on probabilities.

As a patient, you assume that you and your doctor are considering the same situation when you talk about what's in your best interest. But a number of factors make this possibility remote unless the doctor consciously tries to step out of his or her professional role or to bring you into the decision-making process. For one thing, every doctor comes equipped with blinders that have been referred to as *functional bias*. The term describes the predisposition of doctors, as a result of their training and experience, to view any medical problem not only from a medical viewpoint, but from a narrow specialty angle as well.

Generally, doctors are likely to be addressing the matter of survival, which, after all, is the work for which they have trained. Recovery rates and survival rates constitute large parts of their professional reputations. The problem is that a surgeon, an internist, or a radiation therapist may be addressing the same matter but using different perspectives, especially when the medically appropriate treatment for a particular condition hasn't been clearly established. Even when they agree on the diagnosis, their estimates of the odds for success for various forms of treatment may not always coincide. In addition, their assessments of the particular risks and benefits may not match. It's possible that none of their assessments will match your own, even if you have been given all the information available.

THE DOCTOR'S PERSPECTIVE

Physicians generally address medical decisions from the perspective of survival at any cost, and they usually prefer decisions that are likely to provide the greatest chance for survival or recovery, relegating other consequences of these decisions to a lesser status.

The history of the treatment of breast cancer provides an illustration of this approach and the ways in which different doctors may be addressing the same problem, but from separate perspectives. For some years, the leading cause of death from cancer among American women has been breast cancer, from which an estimated 41,000 deaths and 130,000 new cases were expected during the late 1980s, according to *CA—A Cancer Journal for Clinicians*. Given the dimensions of the problem, it is understandable that a physician would employ the procedure believed to offer the best chance of permanent cure. In this country, until well into the 1980s, this best-bet approach for all women was a radical mastectomy or a modified radical mastectomy, both disfiguring operations that include at least the complete removal of the breast and the lymph nodes under the arm on the affected side. The surgeons who performed these operations were addressing the odds of long-term survival.

The nine-year-long National Surgical Adjuvant Breast Project, completed in 1985 under the direction of Dr. Bernard Fisher of the University of Pittsburgh School of Medicine, showed that for women with tumors less than four centimeters (about one and one-half inches) in diameter, lumpectomy (the removal of only the tumor and a margin of tissue around it) and radiation therapy was a course of treatment as good or better in terms of survival than the more extensive total mastectomies then considered by surgeons to be proper standard practice.

As might have been expected, most radiation therapists and medical oncologists have been quite receptive to these newer views of limited surgery. Nevertheless, some cancer surgeons still are not convinced that this most recently recommended procedure is the best approach for ensuring long-term survival. Keep in mind that, with all of their disagreements, what the specialists are still debating is what the rules should be in establishing the best odds for survival.

The Patient's Perspective

Not all patients are prepared to accept the principle of survival at any cost. Dr. David Bergman, who teaches medicine at Stanford University, has noted in the periodical *Emergency Decisions*:

Physicians prefer gambles that yield the greatest good. The problem is, greatest good for whom? Will the physician's assessment that amputation is preferable to limb-sparing because it yields a higher five-year survival rate be in the best interest of the patient who must live those years with a prosthesis? In a situation where a patient or family is asked to endure short-term adverse consequences for the promise of longer survival, but the patient may prefer death [rather than suffer the consequences], the problem becomes compelling.

The case of Alan B. provides a view of the perspective some patients may choose to take.

Alan B., a 73-year-old retired teacher, underwent sigmoidoscopy after his doctor felt an irregular mass just inside the anal opening. The growth was removed, and when the pathology report returned, his doctor told him, "There was a cancer, but the good news is that it is probably confined to the surface. That's a category called Dukes Class A. The bad news is that the cancer is too close to the anal opening to remove a safe margin of tissue without your having to get a colostomy. If we remove the tissue around the growth and give you the colostomy, there is almost a 100 percent chance of your being cured. If we don't, the chances are about 80 percent. You're healthy and active and you'll be around for another ten years at least. I recommend we do the surgery."

After the doctor had explained the procedure and the consequences, Alan said, "I'm seventy-three and I don't want to live the rest of my life wearing a colostomy bag. I'll take my chances."

Alan B. and his doctor viewed the proposed treatment from different perspectives, and arrived at different answers. After the doctor clarified the nature of the problem, Alan decided that his own interests were quite different from the course his doctor recommended. His case illuminates a major principle: Whether doctors agree or disagree on a course of treatment, they are playing by rules that you, as a patient, might need to question. It is possible that none of the doctors' strategies will be suitable in terms of *your* personal, emotional, social, or financial situation. When a doctor recommends surgery, medications, or radiation therapy, for example, it is because he or she believes that this is the best form of treatment in terms of that doctor's goals.

The procedure recommended is the way in which the physician has learned to deal with such problems, and it is likely that the doctor's expectation has been corroborated by his or her personal range of experience. The point is that you as a patient might want to consider not only the rules by which the game is played, but the nature of the game itself.

Decisions are ultimately personal, whether they are made by you or by your doctor. The physician can provide the data base, the odds, and the probabilities for each alternative. You have a right, as a patient, to make sure that your interests, your concerns, and your fears are an important part of the deliberations.

KEEPING THE ODDS IN CONTEXT

Making mistakes in estimating probabilities is a common and human trait. A group of scholars has created a discipline around the attempt to understand the ways in which people's natural thought processes can distort how they think about odds and how they make predictions. These scholars have identified recurring themes in the way that people process information to create their own perception of risks, or *subjective probabilities*. Understanding this tendency is important, because when your doctor's or your own perceptions of risk and success don't match the real odds, the result may be decisions that are inappropriate or even dangerous.

Even when you are able to define your goals, and even if you and the doctor have the same interests, the assessments of your chances by both of you still may be flawed. The fundamental rule in applying statistical principles is to apply them in the appropriate situation. Consider this scenario, based on a problem presented to a group of physicians by David M. Eddy, M.D., a researcher at the Duke University Center for the Study of Health and Clinical Policy.

Linda, 32, came to her doctor concerned about a lump she had found in her breast a few days earlier. After examining her, the doctor said, "Given your age, your physical condition, and your family medical history, I'd say that the odds of your having cancer are less than one in one hundred.

"But let's have a mammogram to check that guess out," the doctor continued. "We won't do a biopsy unless a mammogram shows positive results. According to most authorities, the accuracy of radiologists in correctly identifying cancer in breast tissues is about 80 percent to 90 percent."

Linda's X-ray report came back positive. This meant that Linda's chances of having breast cancer were about (a) 1 percent, (b) 80 percent to 90 percent, (c) somewhere between 1 percent and 90 percent, but closer to 1 percent, (d) somewhere between 1 percent and 90 percent, but closer to 90 percent.

If you chose either (b) or (d), you're in good company. According to Dr. Eddy, the vast majority of the doctors he surveyed estimated that the odds that a patient in Linda's situation had breast cancer were about 75 percent. The trouble is that the doctors were wrong.

Using a calculation known as Bayes' Theorem, a formula that figures into the reckoning the probability of a woman of Linda's age, physical condition, and family history having cancer (1 percent) as well as the accuracy rate of a positive reading in the radiologist's report (85 percent), it can be calculated that the odds that Linda has breast cancer are about 8 percent. Because Linda's life may be at stake, even an 8 percent possibility of cancer may be great enough to warrant the follow-up of an excisional biopsy, the surgical removal of the suspicious mass for microscopic examination.

Because a surgical biopsy of this nature isn't a trivial or an inexpensive procedure, Linda's doctor, had he been more aware of the true odds, might have chosen an intermediate diagnostic step, such as an ultrasound scan (see chapter 6). If an ultrasound image had shown a solid lesion, then Linda would have proceeded directly to a surgical excision. But if the ultrasound image had shown a cystic lesion, then Linda would have had the option of close follow-up after the fluid was withdrawn from the cyst with a syringe and needle. For many medical problems that are less serious or threatening than the possibility of breast cancer, an 8 percent risk may be perfectly reasonable odds to justify continued observation instead of immediate testing.

According to Dr. Eddy, one reason that even experienced physicians may guess wrong about the odds of breast cancer in a case like Linda's is that they fail to take into account the base rate for the group to which Linda belongs. The odds of a false positive reading in the test (15 out of 100) are far greater than the odds that a young woman with Linda's medical history, even with a breast lump, will have breast cancer (1 out of 100). In other words, it's far more likely (15 times as likely) that the test was wrong than it was for Linda to have had cancer. Misperceiving or ignoring the base rate may well be the major error that all people, including physicians, make in dealing with medical statistics.

In assessing the odds and chances that you have a disease, the statistical formula known as Bayes' Theorem takes into account a variety of factors—not only base-rate information and the laws of probability, as we have seen, but the results of tests and new information.

Bayes' Theorem is widely accepted in medical decision-making as a way of balancing what appears to be a common characteristic among decision-makers, including doctors. When people are given new information, they tend to be very conservative. In the face of new information, they are reluctant to change their assessments and tend to seek far more information than they may need for making rational decisions. One result is that far more tests are taken than may be necessary.

Despite the fact that Bayes' Theorem is taught in medical schools, studies have found that physicians tend to make major diagnostic decisions on the basis of their personal experiences rather than on accurate assessments of base rate. This bias is particularly common among specialists, who see patients who have been referred for specific problems. Specialists often tend to have a distorted idea of the prevalence of such problems in the general population—or of the base rate. The problem is that even small errors made in estimating the prevalence of a disease in a particular group of patients result in large mistakes in diagnosing individual patients.

The arithmetic involved in calculating the influence of a base rate may be clearer in a problem that was presented to students and staff members at Harvard Medical School by three researchers who were investigating the ways in which physicians interpret clinical laboratory results.

If a test to detect a disease whose prevalence is $\frac{1}{1000}$ [one person in every thousand tested] has a false positive rate of 5 percent, what is the chance that a person found to have a positive result actually has the disease, assuming you know nothing about the person's symptoms or signs?

(a) 95 percent, (b) 56 percent, (c) 25 percent, (d) 2 percent

Did you choose (a)? Almost half the doctors and medical students did. The *average* answer was 56 percent. However, the correct answer is (d), assuming that the positive tests included everyone who had the disease (as well as the 5 percent who didn't). Fewer than 20 percent of the doctors and medical students tested arrived at that answer.

Here's how it works: A 5 percent false positive rate means that fifty people (5 percent of one thousand) would test positive but would not actually have the disease. Then fifty out of one thousand normal people would be mistakenly identified as having the disease. But the *actual* chance of someone having the disease, remember, is only one in a thousand. So that one person who was correctly identified as having the disease represents only about 2 percent (one out of the fifty-one with positive results) of all of those whose test results were positive. As in Linda's case, the odds *against* having the disease were far greater than the *error* in accuracy in the test. An unfortunate result of this sample situation is that for the one person who gained from having the test, fifty suffered the consequences of false information in a test whose accuracy rate is considered excellent.

All of this may seem somewhat academic, but consider the pressure to test widely for AIDS. Under the best of circumstances, in closely monitored reference laboratories, the predictive accuracy of human immunodeficiency virus (HIV) antibody testing, using a pair of specific tests—the ELISA and the Western blot test—is an impressive 99.9 percent for high-risk groups like male homosexuals, intravenous drug users, prostitutes, or hemophiliacs. In these high-risk groups, where AIDS virus infection is relatively frequent, the likelihood of a false positive test result is very small.

However, for low-risk groups, like female first-time blood donors who have no behavioral risk factors, the likelihood that a positive test is really positive is only 65 percent. If widespread AIDS testing were standard, one of every three such low-risk women with positive blood tests would mistakenly be told that she was infected with the AIDS virus. And this is under the best of circumstances.

In the case of a disease like AIDS, high-risk groups are really those who engage in high-risk behavior. Obviously, there is no clear dividing line between high-risk and low-risk groups. Instead, there is a continuum of risk that is determined by the number of risk factors involved and by the frequency with which the individual engages in high-risk behavior.

The importance of base rate is recognized in a number of maxims that are standard in medical schools: "When you hear hoofbeats, think of horses, not zebras" and "Common things happen most commonly." The problem is that this important statistical principle is contradicted by other maxims that enjoy equal popularity: "A patient is a case of one" and "Statistics are for dead people."

The base rate is what suggests to the doctor that when a young man complains of chest pains and has normal blood pressure, is in good physical condition, and has no family history of heart disease, then a heart attack is not likely to be the cause of the pain. But when a 70-year-old man, even if he is also in good condition, complains of chest pains, he is far more likely than the younger man to have a heart attack.

The Problem with Thinking Big

Many people misperceive base rates because they think in global terms. You'll remember that Linda's base rate was described in terms of *the population to which she belongs.* Some diseases and problems are far more prevalent among specific populations than among the population at large.

Of such diseases, some occur more frequently within groups that adhere to a particular life-style. Smokers are more likely to develop lung cancer than are nonsmokers, for example, and it's far more likely that a physician would consider the possibility of AIDS when treating a young homosexual male, a female prostitute, a hemophiliac, or an intravenous drug user than when examining most other patients. Because behavior can be changed, the risk factors that are associated with particular life-styles or habits—like smoking, poor diet, stress, lack of exercise, and failure to practice safe sex—can be modified, or even canceled. The Framingham Heart Study found that smokers who quit for five years could reduce their risk of stroke to that of the level of nonsmokers.

Nevertheless, some conditions tend to occur in particular ethnic groups or families because of inherited biochemical traits and abnormalities. For example, sickle cell disease is found almost exclusively in African-Americans, and premature heart attacks are much more common in families with inherited defects in cholesterol metabolism. What is consoling is that even in the case of such uncontrollable risk factors, there are usually associated risks that can be controlled to modify the odds.

The accurate determination of base rate for you involves the accurate identification of the population to which you belong. Odds concerning the specific population or group to which you belong are far more meaningful in diagnosing medical problems than are odds for the general population. This is why it's so important to help your doctor diagnose your problems by providing accurate information on both the risk factors that can't be controlled and those that can.

You can help the physician identify the segment of the population to which you belong by bringing to his or her attention the details of your family history, your life-style, and other specific factors that may have a bearing on the identification of the applicable base rate. For the most part, the information that you supply is crucial for determining this base rate. Effective participation in your health care begins by being honest with yourself about the factors that affect your health and by being honest when you report information to a physician.

The Problem with Thinking Small

People are much more likely to misperceive base rates by thinking small than by thinking big. Try this simple arithmetic problem.

A town has two hospitals, both with obstetrical units. In the larger hospital, about 45 babies are born each day, and in the smaller hospital there are about 15 births a day. Overall, at both hospitals, about half the babies born during the course of a year will be boys and half will be girls. Each day, the proportions may vary at each hospital. During the year, in which hospital, if either, will there be more days in which 60 percent or more of the babies born are boys?

(a) the smaller hospital, (b) the larger hospital, (c) the breakdown will be the same

When researchers presented this problem to graduate students, they found that more than half of those who responded thought that the breakdown would be the same for both hospitals. Only one in five students surveyed realized that the smaller hospital will have many more such days—twice as many—than the larger one. By the same token, of course, there will be more days in the smaller hospital when 60 percent or more of the babies born are girls.

Basic statistical principles become clear only after aberrant events. Chance occurrences, freak situations, and atypical streaks of "luck" become diluted in the mass of data gathered over the long run. It's far more likely that distortions will appear in small samples than in large ones. In small samples, freak occurrences may not be sufficiently diluted in the mass of data to permit basic statistical principles to emerge.

Most people recognize the theoretical principle that small samples aren't really representative, but they tend to have trouble applying this principle in everyday real-life situations. This is why, faced with a more skillful opponent in a game of Ping-Pong, many individuals don't realize that they are far more likely to win a game of 15 points than one of 21 points. The weaker player can win by getting enough lucky strokes to balance the better player's skill, and this is far more likely to happen in a short game. By the same token, the chances of an upset are greater in a series of two-out-of-three games than in one of four-out-of-seven.

Because it's so easy to overlook the problem of small-sample distortion in everyday decision-making, most people tend to draw generalizations from individual experiences and unrepresentative data ("I know just what you've got; I had exactly those symptoms once, and it turned out to be a hiatal hernia"). Physicians, too, succumb to the fallacy of small numbers. Some diseases that are common enough in the world of medicine at large arise infrequently in the course of an individual physician's practice, so that the doctor's first-hand contact with them may be limited. Physicians may draw unwarranted inferences from a limited range of experience, and this is especially the case if their experience with a similar-appearing case has been recent or particularly dramatic.

In medicine, diagnostic proficiency is directly related to the range and depth of the doctor's experience with any particular illness. If you're informed that you have a problem and that it is rare or unusual, one that appears serious or that involves a considerable amount of treatment or medication, you might want to ask your doctor the following questions: What is your experience with this problem? Would a consultation be warranted with a doctor who has had more experience with the problem?

The Fallacy of Anecdotal Evidence

The fact that small samples are likely to show distorted odds is the major reason why scientists are reluctant to accept anecdotal evidence based on isolated data or a small number of cases. When testimonials are advanced for "new" or "miracle" cures, such reports are not only subject to the distortion of the small sample (almost always a sample of one), but they usually are provided by people who have knowledge of only the positive side of the experience. Such "evidence" may run counter to the statistical odds. It also bypasses the additional scientific safeguard of the controlled experimental method and observation. Uncle Henry may have recovered from a serious illness after having gone on a bean sprout diet, but the odds that you'll beat cancer by doing the same thing are statistically remote.

Anecdotal "proof" of the efficacy of medical treatment is common. In a widely distributed book first published in London in 1969, and reprinted at least seven times into the 1980s, the author describes his experiences with nephritis, an inflammation, in his only kidney. When the problem failed to respond to any medical treatment, he decided to "experiment" on himself by eating only grapes for 23 days. He wrote, "The outcome . . . was so successful that it can be likened to an absolute miracle! . . . [M]y body had completely cured itself—after all orthodox treatment had failed over a period of about 40 years."

"The experience," he concluded, ". . . proved to me, quite conclusively, that the vast majority of ailing people—whatever the nature of the illness—can be permanently cured through the medium of the ordinary table grape, with the aid, of course, of the mind and the spirit."

To reach this kind of sweeping generalization on the basis of the author's personal experience, to which he refers as an "experiment," is, to say the least, a distortion of scientific method. There is simply no way of establishing cause-and-effect relationships on the basis of such anecdotal data, because the anecdotal data that have been selected may or may not be representative of all of the possible examples.

Anecdotal data is often offered in good faith, by friends, neighbors, or relatives who are anxious to share the perceived benefits of their personal experiences. Anecdotal data often appears in newspapers and magazines because miracle cures are usually deemed newsworthy. The experiences are offered as proof by true believers who are zealous and often generous about wanting to spread what they believe is a revolutionary cure, which we can assume was the case regarding the author of the book on the grape cure.

On the other hand, anecdotal data is also the stock in trade of the quack, who relies on fraud to sell bogus medicines or products to desperate people. A good deal of the anecdotal evidence that may come to your attention is probably a mixture of quackery in the promotion of the product and well-intentioned missionary zeal on the part of converts who believe they have been cured by it.

The Postmortem Fallacy

The cases that are publicized and those that are described in testimonials are likely to result in the distortions brought about by the kind of small-sample thinking described earlier in this chapter. In addition, generalizations based on testimonials or other anecdotal data violate another basic rule of scientific method: They use information selectively and ignore the base rates. This leads to another fallacy in logic that's called *post hoc, ergo propter hoc* (Latin for "after this, therefore because of this") or, sometimes, the postmortem fallacy.

This fallacy is sometimes difficult to identify because the sheer numbers involved may hide the flaw. But 5,000 testimonials from people that Dr. Gesundheit's Elixir cured their colds within a week are no more convincing than is a single claim. The fact is that virtually everybody who has a cold is "cured" within about a week, whether he or she takes the elixir or drinks oceans of chicken soup or does nothing at all. As we have seen, most minor complaints are self-curing.

Studies indicate that people tend to believe that one thing causes another if the two things happen in close sequence. If a patient's symptoms are relieved after a particular treatment, he or she is likely to credit the treatment for the cure. The more frequently the sequence occurs, the stronger the belief that one has caused the other. Oddly, people tend to pay little or no attention to the instances in which the "cure" occurred in the absence of the treatment or the treatment did not result in a cure. Since more than 70 percent of all medical problems are estimated to be self-curing, it appears that physicians get credit for quite a few cures for which they can claim no legitimate credit.

Such observation and "evidence" are almost always anecdotal in nature. As such, conclusions that are drawn from them often run counter to the statistical odds that have been established, simply because the odds are ignored. We are likely to remember vivid or memorable examples of "cures" and to be more influenced by such cases than by the odds or probabilities. For patients, the best protection against this fallacy in estimating relationships between treatment and cure is a healthy skepticism toward anecdotal data in general, including isolated events in one's own experience.

Unfortunately, physicians are as likely to fall victim to the postmortem fallacy as are patients. The American medical establishment is rightfully suspicious of anecdotal evidence and of conclusions that are drawn from such data. However, physicians themselves often demonstrate an unfounded faith in the evidence of small numbers. *Case histories* are an accepted method of illustrating the application of a principle in medicine or therapy, or a way of proposing a hypothesis to be tested. (They also warn about unusual situations and instruct about rare problems.) All too frequently, however, the case histories that appear in professional medical and psychotherapy journals are little more than testimonials by doctors. Just because Dr. Smith used a form of treatment that was followed by his patient's recovery doesn't prove that the treatment cured the patient. In fact, given the overwhelming odds for spontaneous remission—the likelihood that a problem will disappear by itself—it is very possible that there was no relationship at all between the treatment and the patient's recovery. Unfortunately, newspaper accounts often seize upon such case histories, or on preliminary findings that are reported in journals, and publicize them as marvelous cures; quite often, they never materialize, but are nevertheless remembered by those who've read about them.

YOU BELIEVE WHAT YOU REMEMBER

There is a human tendency to generalize from isolated but dramatic cases. Until the mid-1970s, for example, cancer detection clinics reported an apparent lack of interest in cancer screening, despite the periodic announcements of statistics on the incidence of cancer. Suddenly, in the fall of 1974, a surge of applicants barraged the clinics. For several years afterward, appointments at these clinics had to be scheduled months in advance.

The sudden interest in cancer screening had nothing to do with the continuing public relations campaign. What had happened was that the public's attention had been drawn to two dramatic and widely publicized incidents of cancer: the mastectomies, performed 17 days apart, on First Lady Betty Ford and on Happy Rockefeller, the wife of the vice-president-designate. In the spring of 1987, the scenario was repeated when Nancy Reagan underwent a mastectomy.

Advertising professionals and experimental psychologists have long known that our attention is caught not by dry statistics but by concrete, personal stories. We put more faith, misplaced though it may be, in personal tales than we do in far more meaningful statistical base-rate data. Moreover, we remember the stories about people who have what publicists call "name recognition," and often these stories become the basis for our beliefs and attitudes.

The impact such vivid cases have on us is one form of the fallacy that, in estimating odds, is called *availability*. What this means is that if we remember events, we believe that these events occur frequently or are likely to happen again. It's much easier to remember dramatic incidents in which lives were lost than those that involve far more common, but less memorable, causes of death.

Studies done by Paul Slovic, Baruch Fischoff, and Sarah Lichtenstein, of Decision Research, have made it clear that people overestimate the dangers of homicides, fires, airplane accidents, and other highly publicized causes of death and that they underestimate the impact of such traumas as strokes (which are four times as frequent a cause of death as automobile accidents, ten times as frequent as homicides, and almost thirty times as frequent as fire). In 1985, the leading killers, for each 100,000 people, were heart disease (328), cancer (188), and stroke (67). All accidents account for the deaths of only 39 per 100,000, and suicide for 12. Yet because the dramatic causes are publicized so much more often than are such a mundane cause of death as disease, most people have an exaggerated view of the risk of death from accidents and murder. It might be more accurate to state that we tend to underestimate the risks from disease, an unfortunate tendency since many of these risks can be modified by changes in our behavior.

A far more accurate guide than memory in estimating probabilities is the betting record of insurance companies, which base their premiums, for the most part, on actuarial data. It is quite deliberate that the premium rates for accidental dismemberment and death are so much lower than those for whole life insurance or for comprehensive term life insurance.

Personal experience plays a large role in the shaping of subjective probabilities. Studies indicate that people who live on flood plains regularly underestimate the probabilities of floods because they haven't experienced floods in recent memory. The purchase of earthquake insurance increases sharply just after a quake and then decreases as memories fade. One result of such memory-based odds is that most people believe that "it won't happen to me," largely because *it* hasn't happened before. Consequently, many regularly ignore or discount warnings about the dangers of cigarette smoking, or advice about the value of using seat belts.

To some degree, of course, all physicians engage in their own memory searches in diagnosing or in estimating the relative values of alternative courses of treatment, and their personal experiences weigh heavily in their calculations. Such tunnel vision is particularly common among specialists, whose experience is so heavily skewed in their areas of expertise. Their clinical experiences validate their distortions of base rate because their patients usually are referred to them only if the primary physician suspects the kind of problem that the specialist has experience treating. As a result, specialists may easily come to exaggerate the prevalence of those diseases and problems with which they deal frequently, and the efficacy of the treatments they propose, because they may diagnose and treat diseases they suspect are present, based on their misperceptions of base rate, rather than consider alternatives. One protection against the built-in bias of specialists is to consider as wide a range of consultants as possible when you seek advice. Someone who has cancer and has seen a surgeon might consider asking the primary-care physician to suggest an oncologist or a radiation therapist for alternative views on the effectiveness of different treatments.

It's easy to see how this fallacy of availability distorts our thinking about common diseases. To a large number of people—possibly a majority—the diagnosis of cancer is tantamount to a death sentence.

This attitude is understandable, given the number of people who die of cancer, and the likelihood that many of us either knew or had some contact with someone who died of cancer. But this kind of subjective probability doesn't always match the statistical probabilities in the world out there beyond our skins.

Your chances of surviving cancer depend on a number of factors, including the kind of cancer you may have and the stage at which it is detected. For example, your chance of being cured is 93 percent if you have skin cancer, 92 percent if you have thyroid cancer, and 71 percent if you have prostate cancer (and are white). But it is only 13 percent if you have lung cancer, and it is an abysmal 3 percent if you have liver cancer. One obvious practical precaution to take against falling into such mental traps—based on small-scale data retrieval—is simply to discount the personal anecdotes that you'll attract from friends and acquaintances when you have a serious illness. Obtain meaningful statistical data, either from your doctor or from published sources. Begin with a general reference book. Follow up with a more intensive search by asking the reference librarian at your local library for a list of sources on the topic in which you're interested. The medical library in a public hospital (one that is supported by tax funds) or in a public university is usually open to the public, and the librarian may be helpful in finding information. Agencies such as the American Heart Association, the American Cancer Society, the American Lung Association, and the Kidney Foundation have free information available. Look them up in the telephone directory.

Another form of distortion based on availability results from the lack of balance in the ways we get our information. Newspapers and magazines are filled with stories about the prevalence of carcinogens and the dangers of pesticides, additives, or fumigants used to treat foods. As a result, many people are left with the impression that there is no way to protect themselves against cancer and that cancer rates are rising rapidly.

The fact is that, with two major exceptions, cancer rates are not rising, and some are actually falling. The exceptions are cancers related to smoking, especially lung cancer, and melanoma, the potentially fatal skin cancer linked to sun exposure. Fortunately, the major risk factors in both cases can be controlled—lung cancer by quitting smoking and melanoma by avoiding excessive sun exposure.

Every substance presents both benefits and risks. For example, some fumigants used on grains to help prevent the growth of molds have been criticized as being carcinogenic. But the molds they control are usually far more highly carcinogenic. It's important to consider both the benefits and the risks when thinking about every health measure, including the use of substances to treat food or water.

The Self-Fulfilling Prophecy

People are more likely to perceive what they expect to occur than what is actually taking place. This phenomenon is the basis for most sleight-of-hand tricks. Unfortunately, it also accounts for many distorted medical judgments.

Elaine, a 50-year-old woman living on Florida's Gulf Coast, went to her doctor to complain of difficulty breathing and a "lump" she felt in her throat when she played tennis.

"Could it be related to the mango poisoning I had about two weeks ago?" she asked. Mangoes, biologically related to poison ivy, have an oily surface to which many people are allergic.

The doctor brushed the idea aside, asserting that evidence clearly suggested a heart problem. He pointed to the fact that Elaine's electrocardiogram (which records the heart's electrical waves) had been abnormal over the years, and embarked on a series of tests that included a cardiac catheterization and a coronary angiogram—both risky and invasive procedures. The results of the angiogram were negative. There were no signs of blockage in the coronary arteries. Nevertheless, the doctor, who had a local reputation as an expert cardiac diagnostician, refused to abandon the diagnosis, and he prescribed propranolol (Inderal).

After a few weeks, Elaine was depressed and lethargic. She looked up "propranolol" in a reference on prescription drugs and found that these were common side effects of the drug. Elaine stopped using the medication and discovered that her spirits improved. At the next scheduled visit, she told the doctor that she didn't want to take the drug.

The doctor reacted angrily. "If you're not going to follow my orders," he said, "find yourself another doctor."

It was confirmed, later, by other physicians, that Elaine's problem *was*, in fact, a reaction to mangoes. While it was true that her ECGs had never appeared to be entirely normal, there had been no change over time in her tracings, suggesting that these were "normal" for her.

Elaine's doctor had applied two very sound scientific principles. He had looked for horses (the more likely cause of the symptoms) rather than zebras (the relatively remote possibility of mango poisoning). He had also applied the law of *parsimony*, the principle according to which if one explanation can account for several problems, it's far more likely to be accurate than are separate explanations. It is standard medical teaching that if one diagnosis can explain everything that's wrong with a patient, that diagnosis is more likely to be accurate than a series of differentiated diagnoses.

Nevertheless, the doctor made a fundamental error by focusing *only* on the evidence that fit into his scheme and ignoring evidence that ran counter to his preconception. By doing so, he fell into another common error; he assigned undue weight to data that fit into a cause-and-effect relationship, disregarding conflicting data. When faced with additional data that may be of great importance, many physicians will simply ignore or minimize the information if it doesn't fit into their predetermined explanatory schemes. In this case, the doctor brushed aside the information that Elaine had offered about the mango reaction of only two weeks earlier and the even more compelling negative test results, because they did not fit into his causal explanation. The doctor clung to a premature judgment in the face of additional evidence. Elaine was subjected to unneeded tests and treatment, but like many patients, she had the presence of mind to call a halt to the process when it no longer made good sense to her.

The fact is, there *is* an order in events, and many things *are* connected. Nevertheless, we seem to possess a built-in need to discern order, and we'll often find such connections even when they don't exist. Medical doctors, like others, tend to see what they expect to see. So cardiologists might see heart problems where gastroenterologists might see digestive system problems, and surgeons might propose surgical solutions in situations in which endocrinologists might suggest medication. Even in the interpretation of "objective" medical tests such as X rays, or in the analysis of tissue biopsies under the microscope, radiologists and pathologists are likely to find what they are predisposed to find.

On the other hand, as in Elaine's case, doctors may *not* find problems that they don't expect to find. This natural tendency points up your responsibility, as a participant in your health care, to try to give your doctor complete information. Frequently a patient reasons, "I won't say anything to the doctor about this lump, because if she doesn't notice it, it must not be important." This assumption that the doctor will notice everything that's worth noticing is based on false hope and an unfounded faith in the doctor's unlimited powers of observation. Elaine's case also points up the importance of knowing the specifics about your own medical history. If Elaine had been aware of the ECG findings over the years, she might have noted the absence of change and asked appropriate questions. As we noted in chapter 2, *changes* in readings are often far more significant that the actual readings themselves.

Pathologists and radiologists, who must analyze samples when they have no personal knowledge either about the patient or about other facts that may be related to the patient's condition, are particularly aware of the limitations of their information. They welcome clinical data about the patient that tells them where to focus their attention. This additional information suggests specific possibilities to look for that might otherwise have gone unnoticed, and it helps them interpret abnormal or suspicious findings more accurately.

For the patient, this principle of the self-fulfilling prophecy suggests a practical caution in deciding whom to see for a diagnosis. Unless you already know what type of problem is causing your illness, it is probably not a good idea to start off by seeing a specialist, who will more than likely search for the problem he or she expects to find, sometimes ignoring alternative diagnoses. While the specialist may eventually rule out a problem, diagnosis through this sort of process of elimination can be time-consuming and costly.

The restricted vision of doctors whose training and experience predisposes them to focus on a narrow range of diagnostic and therapeutic options suggests that it may be appropriate to seek additional opinions from doctors in other closely related fields, rather than one from another specialist in the same area. We observed earlier that a second opinion itself may be more biased than one might assume, for doctors frequently refer patients to those specialists who share the same philosophy and approach to medical practice, and these col-

leagues are likely to agree on diagnostic or treatment recommendations for that reason alone. Because doctors may refer patients to
specialists who are likely to be as aggressive or conservative as they, a
physician who doesn't believe that his patient really has heart disease
may refer that patient to a cardiologist who is cautious about the use of
an aggressive testing procedure like cardiac catheterization. The physician can satisfy the patient's request for a second opinion while
validating his or her own assessment by choosing a consultant who is
likely to share the same biases.

OTHER QUIRKS AND ILLUSIONS

The tendency to distort probabilities points up the importance of
considering as much relevant information as possible. Yet even when
people are given accurate objective information, problems may arise in
the ways they *process* the information. As a result, the way they perceive
the problem itself may lead to flawed decisions. From studies of the
ways in which people make decisions in the face of complex or overwhelming odds have come a number of principles that help to explain
why people may make irrational decisions even—and, some think,
especially—when their very lives may be at stake.

The Influence of the Presentation

Our thinking about a problem may be significantly influenced by the
way the information is presented. We may selectively magnify or
minimize information in accordance with thought processes that researchers are beginning to identify.

"I have bad news and good news," the doctor tells you. "The bad
news is that we have the results back from the lab, and you do have lung
cancer. The good news is that it's treatable, either with surgery or with
radiation."

After the first shock, you ask about the odds for each type of therapy.

"Well," the doctor says. "Out of 100 people who undergo surgery,
10 die during the operation. Another 22 die during the first year. After
the fifth year, 66 of the 100 will be dead.

"In radiation therapy, nobody dies as a result of the treatment, but 24
die during the first year. By the end of the fifth year, 78 will have died."

Which treatment would you choose?

The scenario from which this dialogue has been adapted was presented by psychologists Amos Tversky and Daniel Kahneman and Harvard radiologist Barbara McNeil to doctors, patients suffering from chronic diseases, and graduate students. The researchers were interested in learning if the way a problem is presented has a bearing on the decision made.

The statistics in this situation, based on real medical data, make it clear that surgery is riskier at the outset because some patients die as a direct result of the surgery, but that the odds for long-term survival are better. On the basis of the presentation that you have just read, more than 40 percent of those questioned opted for radiation.

But let's change the scenario a bit. In the second script, the doctor answers your question by saying:

"Well, with surgery 90 people out of 100 survive the operation, and 68 are alive at the end of the first year. After the fifth year, 34 will be alive.

"With radiation, 76 will be alive at the end of the first year, slightly more than the 68 of those who had surgery. After the fifth year, though, only 22 will be alive, compared with 34 who chose the operation."

Would your choice be the same?

Tversky and Kahneman reported that when the problem was worded in terms of chances of surviving rather than of dying, the number of people who chose radiation was cut in half. They found that when problems are presented in even slightly different ways, people give radically different responses. In a sense, this finding is an extension of the Heisenberg Uncertainty Principle described in chapter 1, which states that it's impossible to observe a situation without causing a change. The corollary of this principle is that you can't ask an absolutely neutral question.

People seem to respond very differently to similar, or even identical, problems depending on how the choices are described and perceived. For example, Tversky and Kahneman found that people think very differently about gains and losses. In a series of experiments in which the risks involved everything from money to lives, they found that if people are offered the choice between a small sure gain and a risky larger gain, they tend to choose the sure thing. But if the same situation is presented in terms of a small sure loss and a larger loss that is possible, though not certain, most people will choose the gamble.

This kind of thinking is clearly illustrated by how people handle volatile movements in the stock market. If a stock goes up 10 points, with a possibility of a larger long-term gain in the future, most people are tempted to take the money and run. If the stock price drops 10 points, most people will hold on to the stock, even with the prospect of greater losses ahead, in an attempt to recover the loss they already have suffered. This behavior is validated by studies which found that investors have more difficulty selling stocks that had losses than stocks that had gains, even though the existing tax code encouraged just the opposite behavior by investors.

Similarly, most physicians and patients are willing to settle for sure, small gains. If a traditional tried-and-true strategy will guarantee such a gain, physicians and patients are reluctant to gamble with procedures that promise the possibility, but not the guarantee, of greater gains.

Moreover, most doctors prefer sure gains, even at the expense of small, sure losses. Dr. David Bergman writes:

> Clinically, this [traditional medical] gambling style can be seen in the decision to choose treatment offering a high likelihood of long life with moderate disability over a procedure with significant mortality but which, if successful, will result in long life without disability.
>
> Physicians prefer a gamble that avoids a possible big loss to the patient, even if it involves many small losses. A physician who gambles thus may order many needless, expensive diagnostic tests (the small losses) to avoid missing an important diagnosis (the big loss).

Staying with a Losing Strategy

All of us seem to share a real reluctance to change, even in the face of evidence that our habits and practices are harmful.

Since 1966, Congress has required tobacco manufacturers to place on every package and carton of cigarettes produced for the domestic market a notice that smoking is dangerous to health. Yet surveys reveal that more than half of the nation's smokers either don't know or don't believe that smoking causes heart attacks. Two out of five claim not to know that it causes 80 percent of all lung cancer.

Moreover, in one study, youngsters at greatest risk—those who already smoke, intend to start, or have relatives or friends who smoke—agreed that "smoking can injure or hurt the body" but consistently overestimated the actual number of their peers who smoke, and downplayed their risks of getting sick from smoking.

Several factors help explain why people slough off or ignore unpleasant information that suggests the need to abandon old habits. These include the dynamics of logic traps, such as availability ("It won't happen to me because it hasn't happened yet") and similarity, a form of small-sample error ("I know lots of healthy smokers"). Perhaps even more important is a principle called *conservation*, which is based on the fact that people have a considerable psychological investment in staying with old beliefs and habits.

We are likely to stay with a losing strategy for a variety of reasons. We believe our luck is bound to change. In addition, we have very different attitudes toward gains and losses, as noted earlier. We may be reluctant to admit defeat. Physicians are frequently reluctant to give up a strategy that is obviously not working, because they may have a large ego investment or they may simply be comfortable with a strategy that has worked in the past. Consider the doctor's refusal in Elaine's case to give up a working diagnosis and a course of treatment, even in the face of test results that appeared to contradict his approach.

Researchers suggest that in the assessment of risk, we also tend to maintain consistently an unrealistic optimism. Even when they recognize the danger, people seem to think that *their* chances of experiencing health and safety problems are smaller than those of other people. One logic trap that may help explain such irrational thinking is a belief pattern informing us that "if I have it, it can't really be serious" or its corollary, "If I have it, it can't be rare, and if it's not rare, it must not be serious." Psychologist John Jemmott of Princeton University and some of his colleagues found that if a disease or a problem is common, those afflicted may downplay its seriousness or even deny its presence altogether.

Jemmott tested 60 college students for a fictitious ailment called TAA deficiency, supposedly an enzyme deficiency affecting the pancreas. Half the students were told they had the disorder and the other half were given a clean bill of health. In addition, half of each group was told that TAA is a rare condition, while the others were informed that it is a common ailment that affects four out of five people.

When the students were asked to rate the severity of the disease, those who thought it was rare rated it as a far more serious problem than did those who thought it was common. Those students who believed that it was a widespread ailment and that they themselves suffered from it minimized its seriousness even more. On the other hand, those students who believed that the condition was rare and therefore thought it to be serious, when informed that they themselves had it, tended to deny the accuracy of the test itself.

People blot out evidence that their own behavior might have caused problems, although they are apt to claim credit for desirable outcomes. Neil Weinstein of Rutgers University found that we are quite willing to acknowledge the role of heredity or environment in explaining our medical problems ("You know, my parents are overweight, so it must be inherited"), perhaps because we see such factors as largely beyond our personal control. If we can blame our high blood pressure on a family history of hypertension, we're innocent victims. But if our high blood pressure was caused by a high-risk life-style that included smoking, overeating, or the overuse of alcohol, then we've been inviting our own problems. It's far more comfortable to deny the risk than to make the change.

SUMMING IT ALL UP

The doctor's perception of what is in your best interest may not always coincide with yours. Physicians are fallible human beings and subject to the same flaws as patients in assessing probabilities, but they also have personal and professional biases. Especially if you see a specialist, the kind of diagnosis and treatment you get is likely to be the kind that the doctor has been trained to recognize and treat.

There are regular patterns in the ways we humans misperceive probabilities. Especially when we are operating under conditions of uncertainty, we perceive odds and risks that are quite different from the statistical odds and risks that can be calculated objectively. Errors in perception result from the following human tendencies on the part of doctor and patient alike:

- Individuals tend to ignore or misperceive the base rate—how likely it is that a particular problem will occur for someone of

their particular age, sex, and race, and with their family history and personal life-style.
- We tend to rely on anecdotal or small-sample evidence.
- We may assume that if one or more things happen in a specific order, one must have caused the other.
- We believe what we remember.
- We see and hear what fits with other elements in our belief systems and we ignore or change the information that contradicts what we believe—or want to believe.

Even when we are given correct information, the way that information is presented may distort our judgment:

- The doctor may address problems and questions that are quite different from the ones that are most important to the patient.
- We tend to believe that rare conditions are more serious than common conditions and that if many others have a particular problem, then it can't be very serious.
- The doctor may be reluctant to give up a hypothesis that seems to explain a problem in a cause-and-effect relationship, even when the medical program being pursued is not successful. Relevant information that the patient provides, or that comes from "objective" sources, may simply be ignored by the doctor if it doesn't fit into the explanation.
- Most of us—and doctors in particular—tend to value small sure gains and are reluctant to gamble for larger gains, but are willing to take chances on greater losses to avoid small, sure losses.

The doctor is likely to continue to know far more than you do about odds in the case of specific medical problems. But the more you know of the traps and fallacies in thinking about odds, the more effectively you can guard against such errors—either on your part or your doctor's.

The Rules of Encounter

4

During a visit to your doctor, both you and your physician act out a general scenario based on an ancient and elaborate set of unwritten rules and rituals. Some of the rules have become so clearly defined and generally accepted by the society in which we live that they have become matters of custom. Others are personal assumptions about behavior that rest largely on the roles that you and your doctor assume and assign to one another. The nature of the relationship, as well as the content and the style of communication, is shaped by the tacit agreement to accept the bounds of the appropriate roles. What happens during the encounter often has as much to do with issues of ego, power, and control as it does with the actualities of your medical care.

Because the quality and tone of your medical care depend to a great extent on how you and your doctor interact, the more you recognize the dynamics of the relationship, the more you can contribute to how you and your doctor negotiate medical decisions.

THE IMPLICIT ROLES OF DOCTOR AND PATIENT

The Doctor's Role

The clinician is the doctor in the role of healer. The clinician's authority, sometimes referred to as *Aesculapian* (after Aesculapius, the Roman god of healing), confers a special status on the physician. Traditionally, Aesculapian authority allows the healer to override and overrule virtually all of a patient's autonomy, even if the patient is an emperor or a president.

The exercise of this authority is bounded by a clear set of expectations and limitations. Physicians are expected to possess knowledge of and expertise in medical matters, and in our society they must undergo licensing and certification examinations to demonstrate this knowledge and skill. Physicians also are expected to adhere to certain standards of moral integrity, and in most societies they take oaths and vows that govern their behavior.

Knowledge, skill, and moral integrity alone still may not be enough to confer Aesculapian authority, for such authority also rests, to a great extent, on an attitude that might be termed charismatic—from the Greek word "charisma," which describes the divinely bestowed gift or power that gives one person authority and influence over another. The aura of charisma, used appropriately, can be a powerful force for healing in the context of the clinical role.

Occasionally a doctor's sense of authority may spill over, inappropriately, into other activities and roles. This confusion of roles is the basis for the frequent pontifications of some physicians on nonmedical subjects and at social gatherings. Even in the course of making medical decisions, the doctor may stray from legitimate areas of medical authority into your private and personal domain. We'll explore, shortly, some of the ways that doctors can trespass outside the realm of their legitimate Aesculapian authority.

The public health doctor doesn't exercise Aesculapian authority because he or she isn't a clinician. Public health doctors can't issue "doctor's orders" to patients. However, by virtue of their official positions they can give orders to control epidemics or to protect the environment. These orders may even have the force of law, especially in emergency situations. Public health doctors may also exercise considerable persuasive powers and informal public authority. Former United States Surgeon General C. Everett Koop was influential in publicizing the health dangers of smoking and the benefits of safe-sex practices in the control of AIDS, and in promoting major public health legislation.

Nevertheless, most people would raise their eyebrows if the surgeon general presumed to issue doctor's orders to them as private individuals. This is usually an authority they grant only to their own physicians.

The medical research doctor is an investigator of medical disease and treatment. The investigator seeks knowledge of disease and treatment even if the knowledge may not be immediately applicable to specific patients. Like the public health doctor, the medical researcher can exercise no Aesculapian authority. Medical investigators can enlist patient volunteers for medical experiments, but they cannot coerce subjects to take part in them, and they can exercise no clinical authority over their subjects. Like the public health doctor, they have no authority to issue doctor's orders in the name of their subjects' health or well-being.

The Patient's Role

Unlike physicians, patients take no oath that defines their duties and obligations. Nevertheless, several sets of implied privileges, obligations, and behaviors can be identified with specific patient roles. Miriam Siegler, a researcher and family counselor, and Dr. Humphry Osmond, a professor of clinical psychiatry at the University of Alabama, have analyzed a number of distinct patient roles that have been described in the literature of sociology and psychiatry.

The sick role, described and named almost a half-century ago by the sociologist Talcott Parsons, is the most obvious of patient roles. Patients must meet two simple criteria to be accorded the treatment and privileges that accompany this category. First, they must truly be sick, and second, they must make a good-faith effort to recover.

Sick individuals are entitled to a number of rights and privileges. They may stay home from work or school and receive special care and attention. Being sick also confers on them the right to complain about aches and pains and about the absence of amenities designed to ease their discomfort—behavior that might normally provoke resentment and annoyance. As the sick person recovers, the privileges and special attentions evaporate, and it's expected that he or she will once again adhere to normal standards of behavior.

The doctor's services are enlisted to help conquer the illness. They may also function to legitimize the sick role, because nobody questions the existence of an illness in the face of a note from the doctor.

A patient may be denied the legitimacy of the sick role, however, if the doctor is unable to identify an illness that would account for the reported symptoms. There are few matters more frustrating for an individual who knows that he or she is sick than to have the complaints dismissed because the doctor can find nothing "really" wrong. Unfortunately, the manifestations of many serious diseases (among them, Lyme disease, multiple sclerosis, hypothyroidism, complex partial seizures, arthritic afflictions, cancers, and even coronary heart disease) may have symptoms that are vague or ill-defined. Moreover, there are natural limitations even to the most accurate of medical tests and technological instruments that are used for identifying disease.

To be denied the legitimacy of the sick role when you're feeling sick is no small matter. The effect is so disorienting that patients frequently express relief when a disease is identified. Not only are previously poorly defined symptoms and complaints explained (and justified) by such a diagnosis, but the identification of an illness, we like to think, means that its treatment and cure will surely follow.

The costs of being denied the sick role go beyond the purely psychological. In order to receive reimbursement from insurance companies or other third-party payers, the physician must certify that a patient's condition meets their criteria for hospital admission or for treatment. Failure to meet these standards may result in the insurance company's refusal to pay.

The criteria for being in the sick role may be fuzzy in some cases, especially for those people with chronic illness or for the elderly. Chronic illness, the degenerative diseases of aging—like arthritis and sensory impairment—or the permanent impairment resulting from an acute illness can create a new state of "normality" for the affected individual. Such people are often considered *impaired* rather than *sick*. This means that they may be relieved of some of their duties and obligations but that they are still expected to cope by being as self-sufficient as possible.

It can be very difficult to determine whether someone has a new problem that has been superimposed on a chronic illness or whether the new symptom is yet another manifestation of the chronic underlying problem. The distinction is more than academic. If the problem is simply a reflection of the old problem, the victim is not entitled to the benefits or privileges of the sick role.

The psych role, in our culture, is assigned not only to the mentally ill, but also to people who are troubled, unhappy, in conflict, unfulfilled, or who may simply be engaged in some sort of psychotherapy, even if it's only for the goal of self-improvement.

Those who have a mental problem that is recognized as a legitimate illness by the medical community, such as schizophrenia, bipolar depression (manic-depressive illness), or Alzheimer's disease, are accorded all of the rights and privileges of the sick role. However, for the vast majority of troubled, unhappy, or conflicted people for whom a clearly medical diagnosis cannot be made, the psych role is a state of medical limbo. Neither their doctors nor others in their lives regard them as sick, and the people around them see no reason to accord them any release from their usual responsibilities. It is generally assumed that such people haven't been able to cope as well as those around them with the stresses and pressures of everyday life.

Others, such as alcoholics, or tobacco or drug abusers, occupy a sort of purgatory—an intermediate or ambiguous medical status. While these problems are defined as disorders in the American Psychiatric Association's *Diagnostic and Statistical Manual,* the prevailing view of society in general is that those who fall into these categories are less victims of disease than they are offenders who brought their problems on themselves.

The sick role and the psych role rest on distinct sets of assumptions and implications. The sick role suggests innocence and an absence of responsibility for the condition; someone who is sick is the victim of a disease, and needs help and support. Few would suggest that sick people are responsible for being sick, even if they are chronic smokers or workaholics or worriers. Fewer still would urge them to "just snap out of it" and get well by exercising willpower. The psych role, on the other hand, implies an absence of a real disease and also implies that the person who has been cast in that role bears the major responsibility for getting well.

Your physician may relegate you to the psych role if he or she can't identify a clearly organic explanation for the reported complaints or symptoms. Usually, such assignment is considered a put-down and an implication that the pain you're suffering isn't "real" pain because "it's all in your mind."

The guinea-pig role refers to those circumstances under which patients are unwittingly subjected to experimentation that is not designed for their personal diagnosis or being used to guide their specific treatment. Scientific trials are perfectly legitimate, of course, but they require voluntary informed participation, with the clear option of dropping out at any point. It is not uncommon, however, for patients to be assigned to the guinea-pig role by doctors who have confused their own clinical and research roles.

Although both the sick role and the guinea-pig role may involve experimentation, from the patient's point of view they are very different. The fundamental difference is that experimentation in the sick role is designed to clarify a diagnosis or to monitor a patient's responses to a proposed course of treatment. It focuses on one goal: to achieve the most accurate diagnosis or the most effective therapeutic results for the individual patient. In contrast, the objective of the researcher is to obtain answers to a problem in which he or she is personally interested, whether or not these answers are useful in the treatment of a particular patient.

Experimentation for research purposes may or may not benefit you as a patient and, in fact, it may even harm you. The doctor who misuses Aesculapian authority to enlist you without your *informed* consent, or even your knowledge, in an experiment that isn't designed to help you directly is violating the first principle of the Hippocratic oath: *First, do no harm.* So, too, is the doctor who knowingly orders unnecessary—and sometimes expensive, uncomfortable, or risky—tests to satisfy his or her curiosity, even when the course of an illness is already under control.

Dr. Eugene Robin of Stanford University Medical School described the case of a man who suffered a major stroke that turned him into "a vegetable without thought, response or movement" as the result of unnecessary, invasive testing. Robin wrote, "This patient was not a victim of bad luck. He was a victim of bad judgment fostered by a medical system that emphasizes diagnosis as an end unto itself, divorced from treatment."

As a patient, you have every right to assume that the experimentation to which you might be subjected is focused on helping to diagnose your own situation or to make judgments about your own particular treatment. It's often very easy for a doctor to blur the distinction between his or her roles as clinician and researcher, and your role as sick patient and experimental subject. This means that you should never hesitate to ask:

- In what way will the results of this test affect my treatment? and
- In what way will this treatment affect my condition?

The answers may make an enormous difference in making your decision.

There's another form of experimentation that ostensibly is directed toward clarifying a patient's diagnosis or treatment but that may not be as useful *for that patient* as it might appear to be. Dr. Robin points out that when a newly devised invasive procedure is introduced into medical practice, the doctors using it go through a learning process. Because the doctors must gradually become proficient in using the procedure, the patients subjected to it at this early point are subjects in an experimental situation that will help the doctors more than it will help the patient. During these early stages, the danger to the patient is highest, and it is likely to decrease as the group—doctors, nurses, technicians—gains experience.

"Patients managed early in the learning phase," writes Robin, "are sacrificed because of relative inexperience. That the sacrifice is not an inevitable consequence of their disease is usually not apparent to the patient or the patient's family."

The risk to the patient in the experimental use of innovative, noninvasive techniques, such as magnetic resonance imagery (MRI) and state-of-the-art scanners, is not as obvious, because the immediate physical risks are not present. However, the technicians who use the machines aren't as proficient as they will be after more practice, and the physicians interpreting the images are not as accurate as they will become with more experience. As a result, the interpretation of images for the earliest patients using these machines is likely to be far less accurate or useful than that for later patients. This hidden risk of inexperience lies behind our advice that you ask about your doctor's experience with any diagnostic or treatment procedure.

The dying role is very different from the other roles we have mentioned, and it is described at length in chapter 8.

You should be aware that in several situations, the implicit role of the patient isn't always clear. If you have a routine checkup, for example, or if you need administrative approval to start a new job or to return to work, you're not sick, but your status still may not be truly neutral in the eyes of the doctor. Most physicians assume that when you make an appointment you are potentially in the sick role until proven otherwise. And because doctors fear the possibility of malpractice suits if they overlook a diagnosis, they will be especially cautious in assigning you a role other than that of a sick patient, actual or potential. From this perspective, every laboratory variation, minor symptomatic complaint, or slight abnormality detected during a physical exam may suggest a series of tests to prove that you are well.

As a patient, you should be concerned with setting limits to such explorations, and later we will offer suggestions for handling such situations and establishing such limits.

SPHERES OF AUTHORITY

Almost every medical decision involves two sets of issues. Some questions are purely medical and technical, and these fall primarily within the realm of the expert, the doctor, who is almost certain to know more about the medical aspects of your problem than you do. But as we have observed, some choices deal primarily with issues of comfort, risk, and cost. These are the choices that are fundamentally yours to make.

The Doctor's Realm

Physicians deal with questions of diagnosis (What is the problem and how can it best be investigated?), of prognosis (What is likely to be the course of the disorder?), and of treatment alternatives. In each of these areas, the doctor will be able to provide you with information, to present alternatives and to offer recommendations. The more questions you ask about odds and outcomes, about the doctor's personal experience and reports in the medical literature, the more information you will have on which to base a rational decision.

The Patient's Realm

The doctor's recommendations will be based, in large part, on technical issues: odds, outcomes, and standards and practices that prevail in the medical community. They will also be based on personal preferences and values that may or may not reflect yours.

As a patient, you have a right to choose between the diagnostic and treatment alternatives that are available to you. You have a right to decide, in effect, what you're willing to pay in discomfort, in personal risk, and in money to get the diagnostic information or the benefits of the proposed treatment. For the most part, although the doctor certainly may recommend one or another, the decisions and choices among the alternatives go well beyond the technical questions that are within the doctor's domain.

Bear in mind that if you forfeit the right to decide, the doctor will almost certainly make the decision for you. Some of the decisions may be irrevocable and some may not be those you might have chosen to make.

Maintaining Your Perspective

We have noted a number of reasons why your doctor's choice might not be yours, including what happens when various specialists evaluate your case from their own very particular perspectives. Despite the differences in their views and approaches, however, almost all physicians have a conservative view of medical decision-making. For the most part, doctors tend to see the central issue as survival, a challenge in which the most desirable goal is the preservation of life at virtually any cost. As a result, most doctors recommend the procedures that are most likely to result in the longest survival, without as much consideration for what they see to be more tangential issues: possible pain or discomfort, disfigurement, loss of function or of independence. Many physicians are far more comfortable talking about survival or life extension—issues that are relatively quantifiable—than about such subjective issues as "quality of life." Nevertheless, it is just such qualitative concerns that may be most important to many patients. Remain aware of these differences.

When Value Judgments Clash

Like you, your doctor has a set of personal preferences and values. Your program and your doctor's program may be based on individual religious convictions or ethical standards of behavior, on individual tolerances for uncertainty or for risk, on personal estimates of whether a given course of treatment is worth its cost, or on idiosyncratic personal preferences. Your doctor almost certainly will offer recommendations that go beyond technical considerations. He or she usually will offer ideas about how much risk you should take or how much discomfort you should be prepared to endure in exchange for the projected benefits.

Many patients are inclined to delegate such decisions to the doctor. Confused and anxious, they prefer to let an expert decide for them. And most doctors are prepared to make these tough decisions. However, keep in mind that these are *personal value judgments* that are in the *patient's realm*, not technical questions that are in the doctor's realm. In these judgments, the doctor is acting not as an expert, but as another individual who has his or her own sets of ethical and personal standards and agendas.

Legally and morally, you have a right to choose among the alternatives presented, to follow or reject your doctor's recommendations, to agree to tests or continued treatment, or to refuse the treatment that has been recommended or ordered. This right to choose rests on a presumption that you are *competent*, a legal, not a medical, term. This means that you are in full possession of your mental faculties and can choose rationally.

There are times when people may not be able to make decisions for themselves: when they are comatose, or when their illness or its treatment prevents them from thinking clearly. Doctors have frequently assumed that they bear the major responsibility for making decisions for the incompetent, and the medical literature is rich in references to the "difficult and lonely tasks" of doctors confronted with making life-and-death decisions for such patients.

Such sentiments are based on a failure to recognize the bounds of legitimate medical responsibility. Patients or families who give up the control of making such value judgments, or doctors who seize control, have confused the realms of technical expertise and personal value judgments. Before you relinquish your control to make decisions, ask yourself: Is this a technical decision in which the doctor's training and experience make him an expert, or is it a value judgment in which I will permit the doctor to substitute his or her personal preferences and wishes for my own?

There is another side to this issue. If a doctor refuses to honor your request to perform an abortion, for example, or to disconnect a respirator, or to prescribe a drug that he or she thinks is useless or dangerous, you have a legal and ethical right to seek another doctor. But you don't have a right to demand that the doctor violate his or her own moral code, any more than the doctor has a right to infringe on your personal preferences or moral imperatives.

THE TRAPPINGS OF MEDICAL AUTHORITY

Issues of power and control influence the exercise of the rights and privileges appropriate to the roles we have been examining.

More than do experts in almost any other field, physicians tend to exercise their expertise in terms of authority. While lawyers, dentists, auto mechanics, or financial consultants are likely to offer advice and make recommendations, the doctor's advice is often couched in the form of doctor's orders. This unilateral exercise of power may be justified, in some situations, by the vital nature of the medical relationship in which the doctor may literally make life-or-death judgments and decisions. For the most part, however, the unequal exercise of power has come to characterize the traditional medical encounter even when urgency or survival is not at issue. The exercise of power itself can overshadow other aspects of the doctor-patient relationship, and it can distort the decision-making process for both parties.

Much of the doctor's authority is enhanced by such devices as the white coat, the stethoscope, and the operating room "greens" and by the use of a special language. Modest as these trappings of authority may be, they confer on the doctor instant recognition of his or her clinical status and the implicit Aesculapian authority to issue doctor's orders.

Aside from such relatively innocuous assertions of authority, doctors also may engage in certain behavior in order to inflate their authority or to protect their territory. Whether such behavior is conscious or unconscious, it tends to distort legitimate doctor-patient roles and communication.

The Uses and Abuses of Medicalese

Frequently, a patient will listen to the doctor's "explanation" of a problem and wish he or she knew what the doctor was talking about.

Certainly "dermatitis" is no more precise than "rash," and "myocardial infarction" doesn't describe a condition more clearly than does "heart attack." And it is difficult to understand why the Greek prefix "osteo-" is often substituted for the equally clear term "bone." Most of us assume that the purpose of arcane medical language is to ensure precise communication in a highly scientific realm, but some medical terms are actually less precise than their everyday English counterparts. In fact, most doctors' use of medicalese when talking to their patients can probably be attributed to custom and habit. Most physicians aren't self-consciously trying to impress their patients with the language. They're simply communicating in the language that they and other physicians use every day.

Nevertheless, there's more than a trace of deliberate elitism in the use of medicalese. If you've read up on your problem and try to discuss it with your doctor in the presumably precise terms that appear in the literature, you may be told with a smile of condescension, "Why don't you just tell me your problem in simple English, without using those fancy terms?"

Sometimes medicalese can be used deliberately to withhold information from patients. Doctors are sometimes afraid that if they admit that they don't have answers, they'll lose the respect of their patients. So, rather than say "I don't know," your doctor may write on medical records or tell you that a condition or complaint is "nonspecific," "atypical," or "idiopathic."

The use of medicalese is also sometimes justified as a way for physicians to avoid alarming their patients. The rationale is that patients may be given more information than they can understand, or more than they can deal with emotionally. A survey of physicians that was reported in the *Journal of the American Medical Association* in May 1989 revealed that the majority of physicians surveyed admitted that they were willing to engage in some form of deception in the name of what *they* perceived to be their patients' welfare. However, surveys have also made it clear that the overwhelming majority of patients want as much information as possible, and surely the use of medicalese only compounds the problem of the inability of patients to comprehend. While patients can't always be expected to understand the technicalities of a diagnosis or a proposed treatment, there are few situations in which the basic elements of either can't be expressed in simple language.

The ability of patients to cope emotionally is a more ambiguous area. However, it should be your decision, not the doctor's, whether to limit the amount of information you are prepared to handle. If you think the doctor is withholding information by using medicalese, you can let him or her know, tactfully, that you expect to be informed, by saying, "I'm having some trouble understanding. Could you tell me exactly what the problem is, in more simple language?"

More often, technical diagnostic labels are used to give the illusion that a doctor thoroughly understands a problem. After all, when an illness is given a specific name, it offers the impression that the doctor has not only identified the problem, but has clear indications of the appropriate course of action.

Here are several simple but effective ways of dealing with medicalese. First, don't pretend that you understand when you don't. It's far more important to know just what your problem may be, or the course of treatment that's being proposed, than it is to admit that you don't understand what the doctor is telling you.

Second, speak up well before you become angry and may provoke an angry reaction. Triggering anger interferes not only with communication, but with your doctor's medical judgment as well. Say with a smile, "Just a minute, doctor. Can you put that in terms that I can understand better?" Or just, "I don't understand." Or, "What does 'lymphocytes' mean?"

Above all, ask questions as a matter of course. Many doctors enjoy the role of teacher.

The Bedside Manner and the Office Visit

Some experts in communication suggest that you can surmise from your first contact with a doctor how willing he or she will be to share medical information and to welcome your sharing the decision-making role. Physicians who seem uneasy about communicating with you or who tend to rush through the office encounter are often poor candidates for properly assessing your own particular needs and respecting your value judgments.

You can sense your doctor's attitude from a myriad of such signals, verbal and nonverbal. The doctor who always stands at your hospital bedside and the doctor who pulls a chair over to the bed to talk with you are giving very different messages about how much power and authority they are willing to share.

Even the doctor's waiting room or office procedures can provide information about the doctor's attitude. Not only is time money, but the control of it is an exercise in power. Consider whether the doctor's scheduling is reasonable in terms of responsible care. Some interviews can be scheduled for a few minutes, if the problem is a simple one that can be handled briefly. Others may require considerable time. In any event, your major questions should be answered to your satisfaction, and, unless you're a nonstop talker, you shouldn't feel that the doctor is rushing you out of the examining room or office to see the next patient. You should expect to leave the office with the sense that you understand what your problem is and how you and the doctor are going to deal with it.

Long waits in the waiting room are another indication of the possible misuse of power and a doctor's possible lack of consideration for his or her patients. From time to time, emergencies do arise, and physicians may be at a hospital or dealing with a walk-in emergency. But in a good office, a receptionist or nurse will try to contact patients in advance, whenever possible, to let them know about a delay. At the very least, the doctor or one of the staff should apologize for a long wait, and if the delay promises to be extended, offer patients the option of rescheduling their appointments.

When you're in the examining room, you should be given the choice of waiting to undress until you have spoken with the doctor about your concerns and complaints. Many people are uncomfortable and feel vulnerable when they are asked to wait in their underwear or are naked in an open-backed paper gown. It's disconcerting, at the least, for a near-naked patient to discuss a problem with a fully dressed doctor. In a situation like this, you might simply indicate to the nurse that you'd prefer to undress after you've spoken with the doctor. Be aware that the cost of asserting your preference may be a chilly response for disrupting the office routine—and implictly defying the doctor's authority.

In many cases, the authoritarian or unilateral exercise of power is also bad medicine. Doctors who do not communicate clearly will have patients who may not understand or follow their medical instructions or advice. This problem is easily compounded, because these doctors are also least likely to check on whether their patients understand the problem and the nature of the proposed treatment. Physicians who fail to respond to questions, or who denigrate patients for asking "foolish" or "ill-informed" questions, convey the attitude that they are more eager to move on to another patient than they are to clear up misunderstandings or confusions.

PLANNING TO PARTICIPATE IN YOUR MEDICAL CARE

There are times when patients may have good reason to give up their right to participate in making medical decisions. For the most part, these situations occur when there's an emergency: when a patient has been in a serious accident, is having a heart attack, or is suffering from another medical or surgical emergency. At these times, the patient isn't in a position to analyze and weigh alternatives or to question details of the proposed treatment. By the same token, when a patient's blood is spurting on an emergency room stretcher, the doctor isn't likely to explain how he or she intends to proceed or to outline alternative measures. In such situations, you as a patient must trust in your choice of doctor or health-care setting, and hope that the best decisions will be made for you.

However, most encounters with doctors don't involve these kinds of emergencies, in which minutes or seconds count. And even in these common nonemergency contacts, you can easily give up control over your own health and your own body by making premature decisions that are suggested, or even "ordered," by your doctor. Some of these decisions may be not only premature, but irrevocable as well.

In most medical encounters, certain pressures make it easy for patients to give up their right to participate in making medical decisions. You can identify and recognize these pressures and resist them or learn to use your own methods to avoid abandoning your legitimate right to participate.

Dealing with the Lopsided Medical Encounter

Let's consider some of the factors that make it unlikely that you and your physician will participate as equals in discussing the issues about which you are both concerned: your health and well-being. Unless you recognize the dynamics of the encounter, you may take one of two unproductive courses of action. You can easily alienate the doctor and thereby interfere with his or her good judgment, or you can succumb to the considerable pressure to accept passively your doctor's recommendations and suggestions.

Alienating the doctor. A 1988 study by psychiatrist Robert Smith and psychologist George Zimny, reported in *Psychosomatics*, provides a glimpse at the kinds of patient behavior that are likely to provoke doctors into annoyance or even anger. The patients that doctors found most troubling were those who threatened the physicians' sense of professional competence and integrity. In fact, patients who were disrespectful or critical were described by the doctors surveyed as even more irritating than those who failed to follow instructions, who were demanding, or who failed to pay their bills.

Clearly, challenging your doctor's recommendations may disrupt an already fragile relationship. A disturbing implication is that it may also be hazardous to your health, because by provoking an emotional response in your physician, you may unwittingly interfere with his or her diagnostic accuracy and the objectivity of treatment decisions.

Part of the exercise of authority involves control of the interview or encounter. Third on the list of patient behaviors that physicians found annoying was that the patient "keeps trying to control our interaction by interrupting, not listening, or changing the subject." Not only did the physicians surveyed assert their need to dominate the encounter, but they resented any resultant expression of anger by the patient. In fact, a patient's anger was number two on the list of objectionable behavior.

Such findings suggest that provoking your doctor is, in addition to being useless, counterproductive in terms of getting what you want or need. The same caution applies in hospitals, when you deal with nurses. You are far more likely to achieve your purposes through negotiation rather than through confrontation (see chapter 5).

The danger of premature closure. The doctor's need to control the interview can compromise the quality of your medical care in a number of ways. His or her control over the interview creates the danger that communication will be closed before you have had a chance to make your concerns and interests clear. Unless you succeed in making them clear to the doctor before he or she stops listening, your physician won't have enough information on which to base an accurate diagnosis or to deal with the matters that bother you.

In chapter 1, we touched on some of the ways that doctors think while diagnosing problems and arriving at decisions. These patterns have a major impact on how you and your doctor interact. You may remember that *physicians generate hypotheses early,* often within minutes, or even seconds, of the opening of the encounter. As a result, information that emerges early has a far greater impact on the direction of the interview than does information that is provided later.

Physicians interrupt frequently, usually to test their hypotheses. The doctor rarely lets the patient develop a story uninterrupted, with the first interruption typically occurring 18 seconds after the start of the conversation. During the bulk of the discussion, the physician will be more concerned with verifying his or her hypotheses by asking questions than with listening to patient-generated comments or questions.

Not all problems in communication come from doctors' attitudes and procedures. Patients' behavior and problems often contribute to problems in the relationship. Patients are likely to bring to the encounter their own physical and emotional problems, which may create static and interfere with the clarity of the communication. They may be in pain or confused about the specifics of the problem. Or, more likely, their own fears and concerns may work to distort the communication. If the doctor suggests mammography or other screening tests, for example, a patient may tell herself, "My God, the doctor thinks I have cancer!" and continue the interview in a state of numb terror. It's all too common for patients to leave a doctor's office with little memory of what was said or with a distorted recollection of the physician's words.

No matter what you do, you're not likely to control the medical encounter, but you can minimize resultant problems by developing a medical agenda. One reason for planning is the likelihood that your specific concerns, your personal preferences, and your value system may not be the same as the doctor's. Unless you make your priorities clear, you can be assured that the doctor will establish a set of priorities for you.

The Medical Agenda

By now, it should be apparent that there are a number of factors that make it virtually impossible for you as a patient to deal with the doctor as an equal on his or her turf. However, there are some steps you can take to enlarge your role in planning the content of the encounter and to increase the chances that your concerns and interests will be taken seriously.

Because the nature of the medical encounter is so heavily weighted with factors that make it easy for you to relinquish your right to participate in your own medical care, planning is important before your visit. A *medical agenda* is simply a general plan for the things you want to tell the doctor, the questions you want to ask the doctor, and the way you will respond to events that occur during the visit, expected and unexpected.

You can't plan for every possibility that's likely to arise, but you can plan general strategies. An agenda is *your* plan for *your* behavior. Planning won't guarantee that the meeting will follow your agenda, because the dialogue is going to be dominated by the doctor. But the agenda will help you to keep in mind those things that are important for you to learn or to say.

The importance of the agenda. In one of the few situations in which medical terminology approaches everyday usage, the patient is said to "present" his or her problem to the physician. The *way* you present the problem will have a good deal to do with what your doctor hears and how he or she chooses to deal with it. On the other hand, the combination of the medical setting, your own state of mind, and the way the doctor informs you of specifics will affect *your* perception of the problem and *your* behavior.

A patient who has just been informed that she has a lump in her breast, a spot on her lung, or an abnormal ECG is under tremendous pressure to *do* something, and to make a decision. As a result, such a patient is likely to accede to whatever course of action the doctor may recommend or — more likely — simply order. The problem is that this is just the time for that patient to step back to reflect on the information, to gather more information, and to consider options and preferences. In most medical problems, a delay of a day or two will have no effect on the course of the disorder or the effectiveness of whatever treatment is chosen. Such a delay, however, will provide the patient with an opportunity to formulate a considered decision.

If you're in such a situation, tell the doctor that you'd like to give the problem some thought and ask him or her to schedule time with you later, in the office or on the phone, to discuss it with you. You also might consider the possibility, after you've thought about the problem, of asking for a consultation with a specialist before making a decision.

Unless you've planned how to deal with both the expected and the unexpected, you may make decisions that you will regret later.

Planning the agenda. Several forms of communication failure may occur in the doctor's office. You may not communicate to the doctor the kinds of things with which you're most concerned. You may misunderstand or distort the advice and information the doctor gives you. You may act precipitously out of fear or uneasiness, or simply because you don't know the options available to you. You may even engage in the kind of behavior that's likely to interfere with the doctor's objective judgment, as we described earlier. The fundamental reason for preparing a medical agenda is to minimize the likelihood of such distortions in your communication with your doctor.

Begin by *clarifying your concerns.* A patient may complain to the doctor about an intermittent but persistent cough. The patient may be worried about the possibility that the cough is a symptom of a major problem—a cancer, or perhaps a serious infection. By simply presenting the symptom, this patient has left the door open for the doctor to follow a different agenda. From the description of the problem alone, the doctor may decide that the problem is a minor one and that the patient wants to alleviate the discomfort of the cough. Prescribing cough syrup will not eliminate the patient's fear of cancer, when what the patient really wanted was the reassurance of a negative chest X ray. Result: a frustrated and annoyed patient. If the patient had said, clearly and directly, "I'm worried about the possibility of cancer," the doctor could have addressed the problem that was of major concern to the patient, even if it was only to offer explanations and reassurance.

Set your priorities. Frequently, you go to the doctor's office with several concerns or problems. You may even have a shopping list of complaints and apprehensions. But presenting such a list is more likely to provoke annoyance than to elicit answers. A disordered or unorganized presentation of your concerns is an invitation to the doctor to choose the one or two that he or she considers the most important, and to ignore the rest. But the one or two that the doctor picks may not include the issue that's most important to you.

Remember that doctors tend to formulate their hypotheses early, on the basis of the information you present. Unless you make your concerns clear early in the encounter, these concerns are likely to be subordinated to the issues that the doctor considers medically significant. In fact, they're even likely to be ignored entirely if they are expressed long after the doctor has formulated one or more hypotheses. Your concerns are even more likely to be brushed aside if they are presented offhandedly or casually: "By the way, doctor, I wanted to mention one other thing." After all, if this issue concerned you so little that it arose "by the way," the doctor is not as likely to give it his or her serious consideration.

Keep in mind that doctors are on schedules. They allot a limited amount of time to you and your problem, and they aren't likely to respond to what appear to be belated and peripheral matters that arise after the "major" issues have been considered.

Prepare for the visit. It may sound, at this point, as if we're comparing the office visit with an audition or a job interview. In some ways, the situations aren't very different. In all three, first impressions are vital, the time allowed for your presentation is limited, and you'll choose how to present your material most effectively. Fortunately, if you mangle your presentation to the doctor, you can always schedule another visit—for a fee, of course.

You can make your office visit more effective by clarifying in your own mind some of the issues that will shape the way the doctor will perceive your problem. Start by making a list of all your concerns and problems. Next, rank these concerns and problems in order of importance to you, from the most important to the least important.

For each problem, consider the aspects that you're most concerned with. Are you seeking relief from the symptom? Assurance that the symptom isn't evidence of a serious underlying problem? Then prune your list to no more than three or four concerns. The shorter the list, the more likely it is that the doctor will deal with the issues to your satisfaction. If your list is too long, you might consider scheduling a second appointment. Trying to cover too long a list is an invitation to the doctor to focus only on those that he or she considers important.

How to Present Your Problems

Developmental psychologists use the term "critical period" to describe the brief period in human—and other animal—development when the infant or child learns to respond to specific stimuli and masters specific skills or attitudes. In some cases, if the right thing doesn't happen at the right time, the ability to respond or learn may be gone forever or it may be impaired. For example, until late childhood, humans can learn to speak a second language without an accent, and after that time, this ability is usually lost forever.

In a sense, the critical period in a medical encounter is the first few seconds. These are likely to constitute the only time when the doctor will be attentive to everything you say. If you've prepared, you'll have a few of your most important concerns ready for presentation. You should present them succinctly and clearly: "Doctor, there are a few things I'm concerned about. First of all, . . ."

If the doctor interrupts with a response to your first concern, you might say, "I'd prefer to just mention my two (or three, or four) concerns first, so you know everything that bothers me." Be specific and concise. Don't provide details at this point, because you're just presenting your agenda items. Briefly, make your priorities clear. One way is to say, "But my major concern is . . ." By repeating your first, and major, concern, you provide clear direction for the doctor.

There are two good reasons for setting out your several concerns at the onset of the discussion. First, as we've noted, you want to be sure that the doctor is focusing on your communication during the few seconds in which you have his or her undivided attention. Second, an apparently unrelated collection of symptoms may be part of a *syndrome*—a group of related symptoms or a pattern of observations that are characteristic of a disease. The connections may not be clear to you, but if the doctor hears them enumerated succinctly, the relationships may suggest a particular problem.

Presenting your problems is only the beginning of the interaction. Your doctor will respond, but not always to the problem as you perceive it. If you believe that you're not getting answers to your questions, or appropriate responses to your concerns, ask clear and direct questions. Dr. Mack Lipkin, Jr., director of the National Task Force on Medical Interviews and an associate professor at New York University Medical School, contends that patients who take the responsibility to get involved can benefit. He says that studies show that when patients are taught to ask forthright questions, they receive better medical care and have better outcomes.

DOCTOR-PATIENT RELATIONSHIPS

If you are to be an effective participant in your health-care decisions, you should be able to recognize the limitations of communication in each relationship or situation, to identify the communication strategies that are likely to be most useful, and to adjust your strategies to achieve what you want and what you need to achieve.

The ways in which you and your doctor communicate and the nature of the negotiation process depend largely on the nature of your problem, the personalities and expectations of both you and your doctor, how you and the doctor perceive your relationship, and the setting in which the encounter takes place.

The Nature of the Problem

People see doctors for all kinds of reasons: for routine insurance examinations, for preemployment or preschool screening, for specific services like immunization, for advice on diet or exercise, or for diagnosis and treatment of a medical problem. As we've seen, doctors and patients assume a number of clearly defined roles that shift with the circumstances of the medical encounter. Each role embodies a code of expectations and behavior, and calls for a specific type of negotiation.

Routine services. When someone who isn't sick visits a doctor for a vaccination or for an examination that is required by an insurance company or an employer, the purpose of the visit is clearly understood by both patient and doctor. Communication problems aren't likely to arise, and the encounter is similar to a commercial transaction. For the most part, the rules of commerce apply, and the patient is actually less a patient than a customer. In such a situation, the customer-patient is likely to be most concerned with the same problems as those involved in a visit to an automobile repair shop: time, convenience, and cost.

However, if a previously unidentified medical problem turns up during the routine service, the customer is quickly transformed into a patient, and new rules apply, with new strategies for negotiation.

Acute illness and emergency services. When you've been in relatively good health, and you develop a symptom that's severe or persistent, you see a doctor as a *patient* rather than as a customer.

When you assume the sick role, you're not likely to have a problem with access to the doctor's office if you have an already established relationship with a specific physician or group of physicians. Most physicians feel a moral responsibility to offer medical assistance to their "established" patients, even if the purpose of the earlier visit was for a routine exam. However, this unspoken moral commitment may be voided if the patient meanwhile has consulted another physician, especially if that physician shares the same specialty or area of practice. Doctors value loyalty on the part of their patients and generally believe that if a patient has been "fickle" by seeing other doctors, then they themselves owe no loyalty to the patient by being available for urgent or emergency care. Physicians often feel no obligation to deal with patients who are not "regulars." If you don't have an established relationship with a doctor, you may have little choice in the case of an emergency situation other than to turn to a walk-in clinic or a hospital emergency room.

As noted, when you see a doctor for an emergency, your communication problems may be magnified and exacerbated. The more severely you're impaired by an accident or an acute illness, the less able you'll be to communicate clearly with the doctor or hear and remember what you're told. Problems are likely to arise not only in your communication about diagnosis, prognosis, and treatment, but in the area of costs and fees as well. When you're acutely ill or seriously injured, you're likely to be far more concerned with getting help than with weighing the costs of tests or treatment—or even asking about them.

For these reasons, when you see a doctor for an acute or emergency condition, it may be useful to have a family member or a friend available to assist you, ask questions, and generally act on your behalf.

Chronic illness and continuing care. If you have a chronic illness or require continuing care for a disability, you're likely to have established a relationship with a doctor. Most of the communication issues will focus on the management of the chronic problems as well as on access to the doctor for treatment of any acute problems that may arise. Someone who is chronically ill or impaired is more likely than the relatively healthy patient to need additional care for acute problems from time to time. Consequently, it's particularly important for those with chronic problems to have a good ongoing relationship with a doctor who can provide easy access to office and hospital services.

Patients who have continuing problems or chronic disabilities are likely to have a very different relationship with their physicians than are generally healthy patients. Because these patients and their doctors see each other more frequently, their relationship tends to be more personal. In addition, well-informed patients who are managing chronic disorders, such as diabetes, Parkinson's disease, cancer, or AIDS, are more likely to keep abreast of the latest research about their problems or may belong to peer support groups in which current information is exchanged. As a result, chronic patients may know as much or more about their particular illness than the primary-care doctors who treat them, unless those doctors happen to be specialists in that particular area. The patient still needs the physician as a healer but not necessarily as a source of definitive information.

Some doctors feel uncomfortable when patients know more about the latest research than they do, because the imbalance threatens an important basis of the doctor's authority—as guardians and dispensers of medical information. When you have a chronic illness and have educated yourself about it, the doctor normally will have one of two legitimate choices: to learn more about the specific illness or to refer you to a specialist or another physician who is more familiar with it. If the doctor refuses to acknowledge his or her limitations in this respect, and if the relationship is strained as a result, you may have no choice but to find another doctor.

Doctors' Personalities and Patients' Expectations

Physicians are like everyone else. They have personalities, strengths and weaknesses that color their occupational roles. Some doctors are open, welcome questions, and try to look at problems and their treatment from a patient's perspective. Other physicians are emotionally distant, discourage participation, and have little empathy with the people they see professionally. Some doctors are flexible and others are authoritarian, but most physicians fall somewhere on the continuum between these extremes. You may have to adapt your communication techniques to fit the particular personality and interactional style of your doctor.

The assertive, flexible physician. This type of doctor feels comfortable listening to the patient and answering questions without being patronizing. Although firm when necessary, he or she respects the patient's point of view and priorities.

This description seems to fit everyone's image of the perfect physician. Nevertheless, many patients are uncomfortable with this type of doctor. Among these are patients who are themselves unsure of their own ability to deal with uncertainty and who need the security of doctor's orders. Such patients may prefer to delegate all decisions and all responsibility to the doctor. For them, the flexible doctor who invites patients to participate in their own medical decisions may appear unsure and indecisive. These patients are likely to feel more comfortable under the care of an authoritarian physician.

The authoritarian physician. A doctor who is authoritarian may be cold and remote or warm and paternalistic (or maternalistic). In either case, this physician is unaccustomed to inviting patient participation in decision-making. We have noted that the very nature of doctoring encourages authoritarianism and that many physicians give orders, not advice, to their patients. Authoritarian doctors may resent being questioned by their patients, because they may perceive any question as a challenge to their expertise, or they may benignly brush aside questions as irrelevant. Physicians in some specialties are particularly susceptible to authoritarian tendencies. Surgeons, for example, are accustomed to giving terse orders in the operating room, where rapid responses can determine the success or failure of a procedure, and often this behavior carries over to their communications with their patients.

Many fine physicians tend to be authoritarian. While such a quality might irritate you, it doesn't necessarily mean that you cannot receive excellent medical care from such doctors. If you have confidence in a physician with authoritarian qualities and if you are assertive and flexible yourself, you can develop communications strategies to help you continue to successfully utilize the doctor's skills. By focusing on the problem itself (a technique that is described later) and by avoiding a direct challenge to the doctor's position or opinion, a knowledgeable and assertive patient often succeeds in establishing a highly satisfactory medical relationship with the authoritarian doctor. Nevertheless, if you are uncomfortable with either the doctor's beliefs or personality, you may want to consider finding another physician.

The influence of beneficence. Regardless of the personality of an individual physician, most doctors accept the concept of medicine as a calling that imposes a moral duty on the practitioner. The American College of Physicians' *Ethics Manual* specifically cites beneficence— the obligation to do good—as a primary moral obligation of physicians. The concept constitutes a large part of the self-image of most physicians. While a degree of cynicism exists in contemporary society about the commitment of doctors to the principle of beneficence, a patient who discounts the impact of an appeal to moral obligation has sacrificed a valuable negotiating tool.

GENERAL RULES FOR EFFECTIVE COMMUNICATION

As we have observed, the medical encounter involves a complex interplay between a large number of factors. Throughout the encounter it is quite likely that your interests and the physician's will not coincide perfectly. Since the meeting will almost certainly be dominated by the physician, you will be faced with five alternatives:

- You can learn to communicate effectively to achieve your goals without antagonizing or alienating the physician.

- You can accept whatever decision your doctor makes on your behalf, at the possible cost of abandoning your self-interest or values.
- You can challenge the physician's authority, at the risk of provoking the physician and interfering with his or her accuracy and objectivity.
- You can ignore the doctor's advice or recommendations, at the risk of reducing the value of the treatment or even of further endangering your health.
- You can find another doctor whose personality, policies, and approaches you prefer.

Why Communication Often Fails

Roger Fisher, who teaches negotiation at Harvard Law School and who directs the Harvard Negotiation Project, and William Ury, the project's associate director, have identified some of the factors that seem to be responsible for failures in negotiating. Among the fundamental reasons for the failure of communication in general, and of negotiation in particular, are two that have particular relevance for medical communication: the tendency of the parties involved to defend their positions rather than focus on their real interests, and their failure to identify criteria for a successful outcome.

Focus on interests, not positions. The Harvard Negotiation Project found that most people fall into the trap of taking a stand that then becomes the focus of the discussion, rather than dealing with the problem at hand and considering options. As a result, interactions often tend to harden positions rather than to encourage flexibility and a willingness to explore alternative ways of solving the problem. Recognizing this tendency can help you develop a strategy for getting what you want or need from medical caregivers.

Let's suppose that you have high blood pressure. The doctor proposes an increasingly potent regimen of medication until the hypertension is under control. You may be wary of medications in general, and you think that you can control the problem with exercise and diet.

Begin with the assumption that the doctor has a greater stake in his or her position than you do in yours. You may legitimately be defending a value preference, but the doctor is protecting his or her professional ego as an Aesculapian healer. It's easy for a physician to interpret any question or criticism as an attack on his or her professional competence. Questioning the doctor's position ("I don't want to take medication, and I'd much rather rely on exercise and diet") is more likely to result in a defensive, or perhaps even an angry, response than in a reflective reconsideration.

It's far more productive to focus on the interest that you share with the doctor: reducing your blood pressure. The immediate issue at hand is to clarify the problem so that the doctor recognizes your concerns. In this way, you will both be addressing the same issue. For example: "I'm very conservative about taking drugs or medications. What would be a reasonable period for me to try exercise and diet first, before we begin a program of medication?"

Another technique is to open up choices before there is a commitment to one approach. Ask the doctor, as the expert, to review for you *all* the options available for reducing blood pressure. Even if you choose an option other than the one the doctor proposes and explain your reasons for doing so, the doctor's position has not been attacked, since that option was chosen from the menu of alternatives the doctor presented as possibilities.

When you focus on your interests and your concerns, the doctor is invited as the expert to help you clarify the problem and to deal with it on your terms.

Clarifying expectations. We humans often judge the success or failure of an approach on the basis of ambiguous and usually unstated expectations. As a result, a doctor may believe that a treatment has been successful because the pain has been alleviated, while the patient may feel that it has been unsuccessful because no permanent cure has been effected. Or the doctor may be satisfied that the patient's life has been saved, while the patient may be bitter because he or she has been left with a permanent disability.

Unless you and the doctor agree in advance on what is expected from any diagnostic or therapeutic intervention, there can be no clear meeting of the minds on which proposed course of action is "better."

You can clarify what might *possibly* happen by asking:

- What options are available?
- What is the best outcome I can reasonably expect for each course of action, and what is the worst that is likely to happen?
- Based on your experience and the literature in the field, how likely is the best or the worst outcome?
- Given my age, condition, and medical history, what do you realistically expect to happen, and how likely is it?

While there is no guarantee that any course of diagnosis or treatment will "work," at least you and the doctor will be sharing the same expectations of what is likely to happen as a result of selecting any option, and the same criteria for knowing whether it is "working." With this accomplished, you'll be better able to work together.

SUMMING IT ALL UP

While their interests and concerns overlap and intersect, doctors and patients function in separate and clearly delineated spheres of authority. The doctor's clinical authority rests on his or her technical knowledge and skills. Consequently, the doctor is in a position to diagnose, to predict the course of an illness, and to recommend a course of treatment. The doctor can spell out the risks and benefits of the various diagnostic and treatment procedures that may be appropriate.

Ultimately, however, it's the patient's prerogative to make value judgments: to choose between the alternatives and to weigh the costs (in discomfort, risk, and money) against the projected benefits. The competent patient has the right to accept or reject any of the proposed alternatives.

Your success in participating in this decision-making process will depend, in large part, on the relationship you establish with your doctor.

Some of the variables that form this relationship may be beyond your direct control, for powerful social assumptions shape roles that are difficult to elude, and the roles also may shift without warning, with a concomitant change in the rules that govern doctor and patient behaviors.

In addition, certain common practices operate to inflate the authority of the doctor and diminish your participation in decision-making. A disproportionate exercise of authority can affect the quality of the health care you receive. If you are alert to such practices, you can take measures to neutralize them or to counteract them so that you can participate effectively in making medical decisions.

In the light of research findings about the ways in which doctors and patients tend to interact, you should prepare a medical agenda before consulting a doctor, to clarify your concerns, to establish your priorities, and to present both information and concerns concisely—and early in the interview. Equally compelling reasons suggest that you also take the time to reflect before acceding to a major course of action that may be recommended or ordered by your physician.

Your relationship with your doctor and with other health care professionals depends to a great extent on a number of factors: the nature of the problem, the personality of the doctor, your own expectations, and the setting in which the encounter takes place. The variables will influence the strategies you'll employ for effective communication.

In all these encounters, it's important to keep in mind that you'll be dealing with medical professionals whose personal egos are interwoven with their professional self-images. A fundamental rule in communicating about medical problems is to focus on your interests and your concerns, and not to defend your own position or to attack that of the doctors or nurses you'll encounter.

5

The Medical Setting

IN THE DOCTOR'S OFFICE

The doctor you'll be consulting most of the time is your *primary-care physician*. This is the rather awkward name that has come to replace the old general term "family doctor." The primary-care physician is the practitioner you're likely to call or visit first when you have a medical problem. He or she may be a family practitioner, an internist (who specializes in diagnosis and general nonsurgical treatment), or a pediatrician (for a child's primary care). Many healthy women at childbearing age see only a gynecologist because they have no other problems. The gynecologist becomes the primary-care physician by default.

People who require attention for a serious or chronic problem may be under the care of a specialist who serves as primary-care physician. For patients who belong to Health Maintenance Organizations (HMOs) or who consult a doctor who belongs to a group practice, primary care may be provided by either a single doctor or a panel of physicians. In most HMOs, patients are expected to see a primary-care physician, who will act in the capacity of a "gatekeeper." The patient is required to consult this doctor first, and authorization must be obtained from him or her before additional services will be rendered, or before an appointment can be made with a specialist.

The primary-care physician has two major functions. The first is to diagnose and treat the many common medical problems, and perhaps some of the uncommon ones if he or she has had the appropriate training and experience. The second is to coordinate care and orchestrate referrals to appropriate specialists and therapists. Your primary-care physician will probably serve as a custodian of your medical records, which include most test results, letters from consultants, and hospital reports, as well as his or her own record of your visits and treatments. This custodial function helps the primary-care physician oversee your medical care and usually allows you central access to your records.

Practice varies widely in terms of what particular services you can expect. Primary-care physicians may perform routine pap smears in the office or may refer patients to a gynecologist. The physician may perform simple blood tests or may refer a patient to a medical laboratory. If you anticipate the need for such routine services as ear-cleaning or insurance examinations, the first meeting is the occasion on which to ask if these will be provided by the doctor. In addition, determine if you should visit the primary-care physician first in the event of a recurring problem for which you may have seen a specialist in the past, or whether you should make an appointment directly with that specialist—a gynecologist or cardiologist, for example.

This first visit is also the time to ask about the doctor's hospital affiliations if you haven't learned this before making the appointment, and to determine whether the doctor will manage care for you in the hospital as your attending physician or will turn your inpatient care over to another doctor.

General Office or Clinic Policies

The first visit is the time to find out about office hours, phone calls, payment policies, and the use of ancillary services. Some typical questions:

- What problems will you normally handle over the phone?
- Is there a particular time of day that you accept or return calls?
- Will your staff file my insurance claim for me or help me fill it out? Will you accept my insurance reimbursement as payment in full?

This is also the time to find out approximately how long you'll have to wait for nonemergency appointments and what to do if an emergency arises during or outside office hours.

Negotiating in the Office

The most promising setting for conducting patient-doctor negotiation is the doctor's office. This is the place in which most doctor-patient relationships are forged. Moreover, of all the places in which medical encounters take place, this is the one in which the patient has the greatest autonomy and the largest menu of medical choices.

Getting to see the doctor. The first order of business, when someone is sick, is to contact the doctor, and often it's not easy to do. The barriers usually consist of the answering service, the receptionist, or the nurse. The way in which you present the problem to one or all of them can determine the ease with which you'll be able to make direct contact with the doctor. The person who answers the phone will generally accept the caller's assessment of the severity of the problem at face value, and it's important for you to avoid minimizing or trivializing your concerns. On the other hand, a patient who gains a reputation for crying wolf—overreacting and overdramatizing problems—faces the danger of losing credibility in the future and may have his or her complaints discounted.

Patients' calls are often screened by a nurse, a practice that may make more efficient use of the doctor's time but that may delay an urgent request for information or advice. If you are suffering from a frightening and potentially dangerous symptom—new chest pains or sudden chest pressures, severe shortness of breath, unremitting abdominal pain, or acute and persisting weakness or numbness on one side of your body, for example—be as calm as you can manage to be, but be persistent in communicating the emergency nature of your call. Tell the nurse or receptionist: "I'm having a [name the severe symptom] right now. Please tell the doctor and let me know what to do. I'll wait here on the phone while you ask."

The doctor with whom you have a relationship will almost always feel a moral obligation to respond to an emergency call for help, even if the problem is outside his or her area of practice. In such a situation, you can tap that sense of moral duty (the beneficence that we mentioned earlier) by conveying your assumption that the doctor *will* do something, even if it's little more than arranging to have another physician see you. Such a question ("What should I/we do?") places the moral burden on the doctor either to act or advise, or be placed in the uncomfortable position of refusing a plea for help.

If you have a problem that's urgent, but not an emergency, you can call to schedule an appointment as soon as possible. In such a situation, you must be prepared to adjust to the doctor's schedule, and you may have to wait a day or more. If you feel a strong sense of urgency, it may be advisable to schedule for the first time available, but ask when you might call back to talk with the doctor or when you should stay available for the doctor's call. If you expect helpful and sympathetic treatment from the staff, it's important to stay calm and to avoid confrontational behavior with the receptionist or nurse.

If you don't already have a relationship with a primary-care doctor—if you have just moved into a new community, for example—access may be a problem. In any case, if you are planning to consult a certain physician for the first time, be aware that the major difficulty for a new patient is usually not so much gaining access to the doctor but gaining access within a reasonable time. Physicians generally believe that their first responsibility is to their established patients, and they tend to be reluctant to postpone visits from such patients to see a newcomer. As a result, you may have to wait days, weeks, or in some communities even months for an appointment, or you may even be told that the doctor is unable to take on additional patients. If the initial appointment you make is scheduled for relatively far in the future, ask what you should do in the event that you get sick before the scheduled time. If you are told that you will have to go to a hospital emergency room, you may want to reconsider your choice of physician. If you are using an HMO, you'll find that most of them have rules for access spelled out in the agreement certificate. Ask the administrator for specifics if the instructions are not clear.

Medical records. As we noted earlier, the primary-care physician is usually the custodian of your medical records. But it can be very helpful for you to keep your own record of selected information, such as current prescriptions, a list of allergies and basic test results, types and dates of vaccinations, and surgical or hospitalization summaries. This is the kind of information that can be invaluable in case of an emergency, when you're traveling or on vacation, or if you change doctors.

The original records belong to the doctor, but you are entitled to the information that they contain. Especially if you intend to travel or to move your residence, ask the office staff to make copies of major notations, ECGs, hospital or surgical reports, and letters from consultants. Some of this information can be extremely useful if you have occasion to see a doctor who isn't familiar with your history. For example, a copy of a previous ECG is a basis for comparison with a current tracing that may appear abnormal; having the record may prevent a marginally indicated hospitalization for symptoms about which your new doctor might be concerned. A record of vaccinations might prevent an unnecessary primary tetanus series if you suffer an injury.

Complaining about office staff. We noted earlier that doctors tend to be sensitive to any behavior that can be construed as criticism of their professional competence. Most physicians tend to regard their office personnel as extensions of their professional selves. Their nurses and receptionists have been selected and trained to project a professional image of medical competence, and criticism of a receptionist may be perceived as tantamount to criticism of the doctor.

When you're faced with a problem that emanates from the doctor's office, it's helpful to refer to another principle that emerged from the Fisher/Ury Harvard Negotiation Project: Separate the problem from the people. In addition to producing a satisfactory solution, effective negotiation improves, or at least doesn't damage, the relationships between the parties.

Suppose you call your doctor and then wait in vain for a return call. You may be convinced that the receptionist hasn't given the doctor the message, and you may tell the doctor so at your next meeting. Perhaps the receptionist *has* been negligent. Or perhaps the doctor was involved in an emergency. Or perhaps another employee took the message and neglected to inform the receptionist. In any case, criticizing the receptionist is more likely to strain your relationship with the doctor than to improve it. In focusing on the problem, you might say, "I've been having trouble getting through to you when I needed some advice." This is a problem that the doctor is likely to be as concerned about as you.

Talking about costs. Medical care is expensive and is getting more expensive all the time. Figures released in 1988 by the Federal Health Care Financing Administration indicate that total health-care spending in the United States was more than $500 billion in 1987 alone and is expected to triple by the year 2000.

Despite the almost universal concern over the expense of health care, physicians and patients rarely discuss costs and fees. Many physicians are uncomfortable about referring to the subject, because talk of money implies that the higher calling of the physician can be reduced to a business. Money matters are usually left to office personnel, who handle billing and collections and help file insurance claims. Doctors in group or institutional practices tend to be even more insulated from financial questions because they are either employees themselves or because they employ business managers to deal with the financial aspect of the practice.

Patients are often reluctant to raise questions about fees and costs, and many assume that their insurance will cover the fees. Some may believe, as many doctors do, that asking questions about money trivializes their medical relationship. The result can be misunderstandings and ill will when the bills arrive.

The best approach is a direct one: "I'm concerned about expenses. Could you give me an idea of what these tests [or this treatment] will cost?" If the doctor is unable to give you an answer, ask him or her to have the business manager or secretary find out.

While large group insurers may be able to negotiate fee schedules with doctors, an attempt by a patient to negotiate price with individual physicians will usually be viewed by the doctor as haggling. It is acceptable, however, to negotiate over the *terms* of payment, and such arrangements should be made in advance, when possible. In order to discuss these issues intelligently, patients should know the terms of their medical insurance policies. The benefits administrator of your company or the doctor's personnel often will help review the specifics of policies. Ask the doctor or, more likely, the business manager, whether your insurance company fee schedule is accepted by the doctor; then, if the information is relevant, inquire about what arrangements you might be able to negotiate for paying the uncovered balances.

Prescriptions: Communicating About Drugs

Many of the highly touted "miracles" of medicine are really advances in the field of pharmacology. The body's biochemical system is regulated and adjusted by chemicals that are produced within the body and by those that are introduced from without. These chemicals can blot out pain, induce sleep, keep you awake, calm you down, make you happy or depressed, and affect how your organs and glands control your body's functions. Used properly, drugs can help in healing, in curing, and in comforting. Used improperly, they can injure and even kill.

Studies reveal a giant chasm between what doctors think they communicate about a prescription drug and the information patients say they are getting. According to two nationwide surveys done for the Food and Drug Administration in early and mid-1983, and reported on by Roger W. Miller, most doctors thought they were giving their patients enough information about prescriptions, but only about one-third of patients said they received enough information about drugs, including possible side effects. Doctors also complained that patients often failed to take medication properly. Seventy-two percent of physicians surveyed reported that patients frequently failed to take all their medicine as needed—but only 7 percent said they actually informed patients of the importance of finishing the entire prescription for those drugs that must be taken in full to be effective, or of refilling the prescription when appropriate. Perhaps the most revealing statistics were that only 2 to 4 percent of the patients said they asked their doctors questions about prescriptions, and only 3 percent asked their pharmacists how much medicine to take, when to take it, and information about refill availability, precautions, or possible side effects.

Such findings are corroborated by other studies. An AMA survey, reported in *American Medical News* in 1984, indicated that only 26 percent of patients received any written instructions from their doctors regarding the use of prescription drugs. A 1988 report from the National Council on Patient Information and Education revealed that half the number of older people who failed to fill their prescriptions or who discontinued medication use didn't even bother to tell the doctor about it.

One conclusion emerges clearly: Doctors and patients are not communicating about the use and abuse of prescription drugs or about the problems that may have caused the failure to use these drugs properly.

Finding out about the drugs prescribed for you. As we have mentioned, some medicine taken at one time of day, for example, may be far more effective than the same medicine taken at another time. Some prescriptions may have adverse, even fatal, effects if they are taken with other drugs or substances.

There are several standard questions that you should ask whenever your doctor prescribes a drug, and it's helpful to write down the answers you receive.

- What is the name of the medication, and what is it supposed to do?
- How will I know if it's working, and how long will it take to see the effects?
- How and when do I take it, and when do I stop using it?
- Are there any foods, drinks, other drugs, or activities that I should avoid when taking it?
- What are the possible side effects, and what should I do if they occur?
- Do you have any written information on the drug?

Ask specific questions if any of the instructions are unclear: Should you take the capsule or tablet whole, or chew it? Will there be a problem if you miss a dose? Does four times a day mean every six hours of the twenty-four, or every four hours from morning until bedtime?

If you take medications frequently, a copy of *Drug Information for the Consumer*, which is prepared by the U.S. Pharmacopeia and published by Consumer Reports Books, or another drug reference would be useful. These references describe the function of prescription drugs, tell when they should and should not be used, and indicate possible side effects.

Not all patients react the same way to medications, and you may have an exaggerated response to a drug, either because you are particularly sensitive or because the initial dosage was too high for you. If you think your reaction may be extreme, hold off on the next dose and contact your doctor for advice.

It's a good idea to keep a record of prescriptions you have filled, with the name, prescription number, and date. Not only will it be useful for your own reference, but it should be shown to any other doctors you may consult.

Brand names versus generics. The pharmaceutical company that developed a drug can receive a patent which gives that company exclusive rights to produce and distribute that medication for 17 years.

This patent is designed to give the developer an opportunity to recoup the costs of development and testing. (A good deal of money is lost in this process of research and development, because many new products are aborted before they have a chance to see the light of day.) When the patent expires, any company can produce the drug under any name it wishes to use—or under the generic name itself.

Your doctor may prescribe by brand name or by generic name. Generics are usually less expensive, and many states mandate that pharmacists use a generic brand unless the doctor specifies a brand name with no substitution permitted. While generics are chemical equivalents of the original brand-name drug, not all generics are equal. Some may be absorbed at a lesser or different rate than the original, and a few manufacturers of generic drugs have been charged with cheating on the ingredients or with submitting fraudulent samples for FDA testing and approval. Some states publish a *negative formulary*, a list of medications for which pharmacists may *not* automatically substitute generics.

Some doctors habitually write a drug's brand name on prescriptions. Others may write brand names because they distrust or are uncertain about the generic substitute. You might ask the doctor if he or she can prescribe a less expensive equivalent that would be as satisfactory as the brand name.

Chapter 7 provides a more detailed discussion of medications.

Clarifying Communications with Your Doctor

There's not very much that you can do to improve a physician's communication skills. But you can take the responsibility for learning what you must know and for clarifying the communication. Ask questions. If you don't understand the answer, don't be afraid to appear ignorant; remember why you are consulting a doctor. Don't just say, "I don't understand." Take the time to be specific, and write down the answers you receive so you can review them later. And be sure to add, as a matter of course, "I think I understand what we've been talking about, but if I have questions later, when is a good time to call you?"

If you're particularly concerned about a forthcoming visit because you're anxious about your problem, because your perception is impaired, or because you anticipate bad news, ask a relative or friend to accompany you to the doctor's office. Then you can review together the conversation you had with the doctor and prepare any additional questions you might want to ask the doctor by telephone.

Asking for a Consultation

A doctor may refer a patient to a specialist to confirm a diagnosis, to perform a procedure, or for a variety of other reasons. There are also times when a patient asks for a referral to a specialist, and fundamentally these occasions fall into two categories:

- You may want to continue under the care of your own doctor, but you want reassurance that the current or proposed diagnosis or treatment program is appropriate.
- You may prefer to be under the care of another doctor because you are unhappy with your current medical care or because you think a specialist would be more competent in handling your case.

The second situation can constitute one of the most sensitive areas in the doctor-patient relationship. A request for a consultation by a patient can be humiliating for the doctor, especially if the physician suspects that the patient is unhappy with his or her care. Those doctors who are emotionally insecure or have an unrealistic assessment of their competence might react to such a request with anger or shame, and this may rupture the relationship between patient and doctor. How should you proceed in such a delicate negotiation?

It's a good idea to avoid creating antagonism, even if you intend to break off your relationship with the doctor you have been consulting. Many specialists won't see self-referred patients, and others may call the primary doctor as a matter of course, in order to get background information, which may include the doctor's opinion of you as a patient. Unless you are certain that you want to leave the primary-care doctor, it usually isn't difficult to affirm your confidence in him or her and point to another source for the request ("My daughter says she'll be more comfortable with my care if this particular procedure were handled by a specialist").

Most doctors will accede to a request for a referral. If a doctor refuses, you may try to contact a specialist directly, especially one with whom you may have had previous experience. If the specialist you want to see insists on a referral, you may have to find another primary-care physician and begin the process again.

DEALING WITH CONSULTANTS

When the primary-care physician refers a patient to a consultant, the relationship between the patient and the consulting physician may be ambiguous. While the referring physician is clearly acting on the patient's behalf, it isn't always clear whether the consultant is answerable to the patient or to the referring physician.

When you are referred to a consultant, ask your doctor the purpose of the consultation. If the consultant has been asked to provide diagnostic data or to perform an independent assessment, then your primary-care physician should retain full responsibility for your care.

On the other hand, a consultant may be asked to manage a patient's problem jointly with the referring physician or may even be asked to assume total medical authority, becoming, in effect, the primary-care physician. Unless the lines of responsibility are clearly established, you may not know who is responsible for supervising your medical care, and there is a potential for failures in communication. When you are referred to a specialist for anything more than a diagnosis, it's advisable to ask the referring doctor to define the scope of the consultant's responsibility.

The *Ethics Manual* of the American College of Physicians stresses the paramount nature of the patient's welfare in the consultation process. However, the manual also stresses the importance of maintaining collegial relations between the referring and the consulting physicians, and on occasion, the two sets of obligations may conflict. The consultant may believe that he or she should manage the patient's care, or the patient may simply prefer to have the problem handled by the consultant as a primary-care physician.

In the latter case, the consultant may have a conflict of interest: whether to act in accordance with the patient's preference or avoid alienating a continuing source of referral business. If you prefer to have a consultant take over the management of the problem for which you were referred, you should be open about how you feel and ask the consultant: "Do you think I would be better off having you manage my care for this problem? Would you agree to take over my case?"

If the consultant agrees, be prepared to take the initiative with the referring doctor by suggesting that it would be easier for you to deal with just one doctor for this particular problem. Before you act to transfer responsibility, remember that such a move may seriously damage your relationship with the referring physician, and then decide which relationship is more important for you.

Another, and a clearly uncomfortable, situation may arise when a consultant takes the initiative in ordering tests and prescribing treatment without the consent of either the referring doctor or the patient. For example, a gastroenterologist consulted for abdominal pressure may legitimately suggest to either the patient or the referring doctor that the specific symptom may be a manifestation of a heart problem. However, it would be inappropriate professional behavior if the consultant unilaterally scheduled a stress test or referred the patient to a cardiologist. Aside from the issue of ambiguous lines of responsibility, such behavior creates the potential for fragmented care for the patient.

As a rule of thumb, if you have questions about the actions of any consultant, communicate your concerns to your primary-care physician.

THE EMERGENCY ROOM AND THE WALK-IN CLINIC

Some healthy people determine that they don't need a continuing-care relationship with a doctor and use a walk-in clinic or a hospital emergency room for episodic urgent care. Unless there's no alternative, we don't recommend this as a matter of course, though being familiar with how these facilities operate is an asset when you do need to take advantage of their services.

The major advantage of such settings is easy access; both kinds of facilities are designed for the examination and treatment of patients without prior appointments. Because patient flow is unpredictable, a patient may be able to consult a doctor almost immediately during quiet periods but may have to wait up to several hours if the facility is busy. Generally the time available for a particular service is not a limiting factor, because there is no preset schedule. If the doctor takes more time with one person, the next patient just has to wait longer.

Walk-in clinics usually operate on a first-come, first-served basis. As a result, for those with relatively minor problems, attention at a walk-in clinic generally involves a much shorter wait than that at a hospital emergency room.

There are some differences between walk-in clinics (known formally as free-standing emergency centers—or emergicenters—because they are not housed in hospitals or on hospital grounds) and emergency rooms in hospitals. For the most part, patients who visit walk-in clinics aren't as critically ill or injured as those who go to, or are taken to, hospital emergency rooms. As a result of the wider range of severity in problems handled by emergency rooms, their personnel usually adhere to a policy of *triage,* by which the severity of medical problems is assessed and a priority order for their treatment is established. Patients with critical or severe problems, whose treatment is the most time-consuming, are seen before those with minor problems. Given this situation, those with less serious complaints may have to wait hours, even though their care is less demanding than that of the seriously ill patient.

Once you're being treated in the emergency room, don't expect any personal communication beyond that which is necessary for your medical care. The pressures that result from patients waiting, the emergency status of many of the cases, and the generally impersonal nature of the ER itself discourage the patient's participation in his or her medical care.

It's worth the effort to plan ahead for a time when you may need the services of an emergency room—if you can't reach your doctor, for example, or if you need an ambulance for instant transportation to a medical facility. First, be sure you know the proper telephone number to call. Many communities now have a central 911 number for emergencies, while in others you must call the hospital itself or a local emergency service. If you have a primary-care physician, if possible call that doctor first in an emergency. The doctor may meet you at the emergency room or alert the emergency room doctors and nurses that you're coming, so that the personnel can be prepared for the tests or treatment you may need.

If you want your own doctor to take care of you when you need to be admitted to the hospital, choose an ER at the hospital with which he or she is affiliated. If you have a choice, check out the local hospitals, because not all emergency rooms are equal. Some smaller hospitals may not even have an emergency room, while others may have facilities that aren't open at night. Even those that are open 24 hours a day may not be staffed full-time, a possibility that would require a time-consuming call to a doctor who is on call. Some emergency rooms are staffed by board-certified emergency physicians, others by newer doctors who have not yet built up a practice and who are on call or moonlight at an ER. Some facilities have qualified surgeons, cardiologists, anesthesiologists, and pediatricians available, while others may not.

If your local ambulance or rescue service has a policy of taking its cases to the nearest qualified facility, you may not be given a choice of emergency rooms. If you do have a choice, it may pay to travel a little farther to reach an emergency room with superior facilities or staff.

Treatment in a walk-in clinic tends to be more expensive than the same care rendered in doctors' offices, and in an emergency room it's likely to be even more expensive. In addition, neither facility offers the kind of follow-up or the continuity of care that you can expect from a physician with whom you have a permanent relationship. Do use an emergency room for real emergency illnesses or accidents, but, if you have a choice, don't use it for primary health care.

IN THE HOSPITAL

Confinement in a hospital is almost always a highly stressful experience. Added to your worries about the course of the illness or injury itself is the sense of dependency and loss of autonomy that's usually inevitable in such a situation. Patients, transported into an alien atmosphere, are required to accept virtually total, and sometimes arbitrary, control by hospital personnel who intrude on their privacy without warning, who do unexpected and usually unexplained things to them as a matter of course, and who often seem more interested in the tasks being performed than in the health or comfort of the patient. The experience can be confusing and frightening.

While room for actual negotiation is somewhat limited in the hospital, there is a good deal that you can do to understand and, to some degree, control what is happening.

Admission

The first evidence of a hospital patient's loss of autonomy becomes clear even before the moment of admission. You can't admit yourself to a hospital, no matter how sick you may be. Furthermore, depending on the circumstances, your doctor may not be able to admit you to the hospital of your choice, or even to any hospital at all, for doctors may admit patients only to hospitals in which they have applied for and been granted admitting privileges.

As we noted, when you visit your primary-care doctor's office for the first time, be sure to ask where he or she maintains hospital privileges, and if there is no access to the hospital of your choice, you may need to reassess the physician or the hospital. For enrollees of HMOs or Preferred Provider Organizations (PPOs), choices of hospitals are limited, and potential subscribers should decide if the choices are acceptable to them before they enroll.

At the hospital, the admitting doctor may or may not be the one who will manage your case. If your personal physician puts you into a community hospital where he or she maintains staff privileges, then continuity of doctor's care from the office to the hospital bed usually follows. If you don't have a personal physician who has privileges to use the hospital, then your case will be assigned to a doctor who is on call to take newly admitted patients. If you've been admitted after being assessed in an outpatient clinic of a teaching hospital or, in most hospitals, in the emergency room, then the responsibility for your care is usually given to doctors who are managing the specific patient unit to which you are assigned.

If your own doctor has privileges to practice at the hospital, the emergency room doctor usually coordinates an admission to that doctor's group of patients, or "service." However, unless the emergency room or admitting doctor knows that you have a personal physician who will manage your case, you may end up "on the service" of a stranger. It's important that you alert the clerical staff, the nurses, and the doctors to the fact that you have a personal physician who can assume responsibility for your hospital care.

Enlisting an Advocate

When you're in a hospital, you're likely to be weak, frightened, and intimidated. In short, you may not be in any condition to follow the advice that you receive. Yet this is precisely the time for you to know which tests and procedures to accept and which to question or refuse;

which forms to sign and which to think about signing; how to make your needs known without antagonizing the nurses; and how to deal with consultants. In short, this is the time to lean on someone who can do many of these things for you and who can advise you on what to do in his or her absence.

When you prepare to go to a hospital, enlist an advocate—a spouse, parent, child, or friend—who will act on your behalf. Unless your primary-care doctor also happens to be a close friend, you need someone who can spend time with you in the hospital, discussing medication and treatment options with the hospital staff, seeing to it that you are as comfortable as possible, and generally representing your interests. Hospitals today are hectic, often understaffed places and unless you have such an advocate discreetly negotiating for you, you are especially vulnerable to the mistakes and possibly neglect that take place in even some of the most reputable facilities. If possible, choose someone who is assertive without being aggressive. However, having an imperfect advocate is better than trying to navigate your way through the hospital on your own. Nurses are sometimes resentful of "outsiders" who represent the patient, so if your condition permits it, decide what matters you can handle and what should be assigned to the advocate.

Hospital Orders

The first task in making sense of the hospital confinement is to identify who's in charge of your care and who will be writing the orders—the diagnostic and treatment plan. The orders are the written instructions on your chart that specify which tests are to be done and when, how you are to be monitored, which doctors may be consulted, which medications or treatments will be administered and how often, and what restrictions apply to your activity and your diet. The doctor who writes the daily orders is, in effect, writing the script for your treatment in the hospital.

The person ultimately responsible for your overall care is your *attending physician*. If you are admitted to a community hospital by your regular doctor, that doctor also will serve as your attending physician. In a large institution such as a university teaching hospital, the admitting doctor may not be your attending physician. In such a facility, you may be assigned to the service of one of the faculty doctors whose job is to oversee a group of physicians-in-training for a specified period of time. Although nominally in charge, the attending physician at a teaching hospital functions more like a general at headquarters. He or she may supervise your care but may not see you every day, and may not even write the orders.

In a community hospital or other nonteaching hospital, the attending physician will probably write the orders. In a university teaching hospital, the orders may be written by an intern recently out of medical school, a resident who is training for a specialty, or sometimes even by a closely supervised medical student. Unless you know who is actually authorizing the tests and medications, you can waste time and effort by appealing to a doctor who may have little practical authority to do what you want. If you are in a teaching hospital with *house staff* (interns and residents), the multiple lines of responsibility can be very confusing.

In addition, considerable discretion is given to the nursing staff in deciding which medicines you may receive, and when. Doctors often write orders specifying that medications, treatments, or even certain tests are to be given on a *p.r.n.* (*pro re nata*) basis, meaning "as circumstances require," or in effect, "at the discretion of the nurse." Such delegated authority may include decisions about whether a patient should be walking, what kinds of food are to be ordered, when a patient should be physically restrained, whether to insert a catheter into the bladder to drain the urine, whether to have blood drawn to test for infection, and when to administer powerful heart rhythm, breathing, or sedative medications, and at what dosage.

When you are admitted to a hospital, especially a large institution or a teaching hospital, you should learn the chain of command. Either you or a relative or friend should ask the admitting doctor, the admitting department personnel, the nurse in the patient unit, or the intern or resident:

- Who is the attending physician?
- Who will be writing the daily orders?
- Who will be making the decisions about tests and treatments?
- To whom should we direct our questions?

If you're going to a hospital for a surgical or other invasive procedure, ask your doctor who will be performing the procedure and who will administer the anesthesia. Also ask who will be in charge of your care once the procedure has been done: the primary-care physician, the surgeon or other specialist—or someone else.

To be sure that you and your visitors are clear about the lines of authority, write down the answers to these and similar questions and keep them handy. In any event, since you may be treated by a number of physicians, you should get to know each by name. Ask each of them for a professional card or ask them to write down their names and their specialties. In most hospitals, doctors wear name tags, as do nurses and technicians. (So do medical students, but instead of "M.D." or "Dr.," their tags identify them as students, with a number signifying their year of medical school.) It's easy to read the name tags when these people are in your room, but if you want to ask the nurse to call a doctor, it makes for smoother relations if you can refer to him or her by name instead of having to use a description like "the thin, balding one with the mustache."

Getting Information

A hospital can sometimes be a "black hole" that gobbles huge masses of information but from which little escapes to enlighten patients or their anxious families.

Part of the problem is that patients are often in too poor a state of mind either to absorb or to transmit details about what is happening. Another part is that many people who work in hospitals believe that their tasks are simply to provide medical services, not to communicate with the recipients of the services or their representatives. Sometimes, nurses and doctors other than the attending physician are concerned that they might be seen as usurping the attending doctor's prerogative by answering questions about a patient's prognosis, condition, or treatment.

Knowing the lines of responsibility helps you and your advocate to know *whom* to ask for information. It's also important to know *how* and *when* to ask. Let the attending physician or the resident or intern who is actually handling the case know that you expect to be kept informed about your tests and treatments, and find out when is the most convenient time to discuss these and receive reports. The *Patient's Bill of Rights*, drawn up by the American Hospital Association in 1973 and distributed in many hospitals, proclaims the right of the patient or family "to obtain . . . complete current information concerning his diagnosis, treatment, and prognosis in terms the patient can be reasonably expected to understand."

Visiting hours may not coincide with the times that the attending physician is available in the hospital, so it might be difficult for family members to talk with the doctor. One way around this problem is to ask the doctor to make a quick call to the family from the patient's bedside telephone during rounds. Not only is this a convenient time for most doctors, but they usually are not as pressured as they are during office hours because their patients are not as tightly scheduled. Doctors tend to make their rounds at about the same time of day, except for weekends, so be sure that the family keeps the line open and that there's someone at home to receive the doctor's call.

The problems of getting information increase with the number of specialists who have been called in as consultants. As we have noted, consultants frequently act independently if they are enlisted to perform specific procedures. When this happens in a hospital, the lines of responsibility may become confused. To minimize frustrations in getting information from various doctors, try to clarify with the primary decision-maker—the attending doctor or the doctor actually writing the orders—what the responsibility of the consultants will be. If it's to render an opinion or to confirm a diagnosis, the consultant will probably report directly to your attending physician or to the doctor responsible for the orders. Many will answer your questions. Other consultants may actually refuse to talk to you, although you'll be paying their bill, and will refer you to the attending doctor or the resident physician for information. If the specialist has been called in specifically to perform an operation, you may be transferred to the specialist's care, and he or she will act as your attending physician. Occasionally, the function of the specialist isn't entirely clear, and you may be left unsure about who has the authority to order additional tests or treatment.

Your attending physician should let you know if a consultant has been called in. If you haven't already been told by your attending physician, make sure you learn the consultant's name (ask for a business card) and the reason the consultant has been called to examine you. Ask specifically:

- What's the reason my doctor asked you to see me?
- When will you be giving your report?
- Will you be discussing your findings with me, or shall I get the information from Dr. [your attending physician]?

Asking Questions to Avoid Mistakes

We have noted that despite their rules and regulations, and despite their general efficiency, hospital staffs make mistakes. These can range from the simply annoying, like the repetition of a test that was just performed, to the serious, like being given the wrong medication. Operations have even been performed on the wrong patient; usually the victims were so certain that the doctors and the hospital knew what they were doing that they never questioned what was happening.

To keep informed about what's going on, you need an agenda in the hospital, just as you needed one in the doctor's office. The hospital agenda differs from the one in the office in that when you're in a hospital, the most important issue has already been decided: You *need* hospital services, either because you require a diagnostic or treatment procedure that's too complex or too risky to be performed in an office or a clinic, or because your condition calls for special care and monitoring. In fact, many of the specific items on the hospital agenda have also been decided in advance. What is most important for you is to find out the details of that agenda and to know what is planned for you, not only in general, but on a day-to-day basis. A major reason for becoming involved in your health care is that if you know what's going on, you'll be in a far better position to avoid the mistakes that happen in hospitals. In addition, the more you know about what's going to happen, the less anxious you are likely to be.

Here are some questions you should ask, followed by the reasons for asking them.

- What *tests or procedures* will I be having, and when?
- Are there any special *instructions* I should follow about eating or drinking?

Many of the tests and some of the procedures may be performed early in the morning before the doctors arrive, so it's a good idea to ask, during the doctor's visit, what is planned or scheduled for the following day. One frequent problem in hospitals is that of the many tests performed, some may duplicate tests you've already had. If you think you're getting too many tests, ask your doctor why they are all needed. The doctor may have written a "standing order" for certain tests to be taken each day and then have forgotten that the order was written. Problems can also occur when certain tests and procedures must be done before you eat or drink anything, and the breakfast tray is delivered inadvertently. This kind of lack of coordination between separate departments is not unusual, and in order to avoid the cancellation of needed tests, it's best to ask specifically about the conditions under which each test is to be taken.

Tests and many procedures, like blood transfusions and certain kinds of therapies, are ordered from the specific departments involved, with the recipient identified by his or her name and the room and bed numbers. It's particularly easy for mistakes to happen under these circumstances, and you've probably heard about patients getting tests or procedures that were meant for someone else. The more you know about your schedule, the less likely you are to accept a test or treatment that isn't meant for you. If you think the technician is in your room by mistake, don't accept the test or treatment until you've asked him or her to check with your doctor or the nurse.

- What *medications* are you ordering? How *often* will I get them?
- May I get a copy of my *medication schedule* from the nurse—and would you write that in the orders?

There are several reasons for you to have a record. First, some medications may be offered by the staff almost routinely, whether you need them or not. Or you may suspect that you are experiencing side effects from some of the medications or their combinations. If you have a record of what you are getting, when you talk to the doctor you can raise questions about the purpose of each medication and its possible adverse effects. This is important because if more than one doctor is prescribing medication, and neither bothers to check what the other has prescribed, undesirable drug interactions may occur.

Certain drugs act in combination—for example, an antinausea drug administered even only once in conjunction with other powerful medications may cause severe problems. In addition, don't leave it to your doctor to remember your allergies to certain drugs; most hospitals will provide a permanent warning in the form of a bracelet or other identification for you to wear, but you must alert them first to do so.

Another reason for knowing your medication schedule is to review it for information on how often the doses are to be administered.

More important, in an institution as large and busy as a hospital, mistakes occur with medications, as we noted. Nurses might bring you someone else's medication, or the busy pharmacist may have misread the order. When you are given a medication that you don't recognize, ask what it is and check your list. If there is an apparent discrepancy between what is on the list and what is actually brought to you, *don't take the medication* until you've checked with the nurse or the doctor. You have a legal and ethical right to refuse any medication or treatment. Moreover, mistakes occur rather frequently in billing for medications. If you keep your own record, you can review the hospital charges after you get home, if this becomes necessary.

Testing and hospitals. In the doctor's office, unless the doctor wants to test you then and there, it's you who decides *when* to have the test, and you who presents yourself to the lab or at the consultant's office. If you're not feeling well, you can cancel or reschedule your test. You may even decide not to go for the test if you think it's inappropriate or unnecessary.

In the hospital, a good deal of this control evaporates. The laboratory technicians who perform your tests come in without invitation; they draw blood without asking and without notice. Orderlies often appear with no warning to wheel you to the X-ray department. Your breakfast is brought at the hospital's convenience—and may disappear while you're out having a test somewhere. In general, you're an object to be poked, prodded, and jabbed.

More often than not, you won't be informed what's happening or when it's to happen. Tests will be ordered without your knowledge, and you will generally not be told what they're for. Frequently, nobody will bother to tell you some of the unpleasant things that may happen to you before, during, or after some of these tests.

Complaints are not welcome in the hospital, and they may bring on your head the wrath of the institution. You may be told that you can ask questions only when your own doctor comes in. Nevertheless, you should remember that you have the right—legally and ethically—to know what is happening to you. Keep in mind that you or your insurance company is going to pay for the tests, and that it's you who will bear the consequences of decisions, good or bad. You can maintain some control and get information by asking the questions on the preceding pages about tests, procedures, preparations, and precautions.

Iatrogenic disease. The word "iatrogenic" comes from the Greek for "physician" and means "physician-produced." As the number of doctors involved in your care increases, the likelihood of iatrogenic complications increases as well.

Iatrogenesis is a major problem in hospitals. Numbers of studies document the high probability of your contracting an illness in the hospital, one you didn't have when you were admitted. In fact, in his book, *Matters of Life and Death*, Eugene Robin writes about "iatroepidemics," or errors that are built into the system. What he means is that some procedures that are generally accepted in medicine may harm or kill patients, more or less systematically. It's becoming clear that some standard diagnostic procedures in hospitals have become major causes of iatrogenic problems. And the more medical tests you take, the greater is your chance of suffering from a problem that's caused by the tests themselves.

Time is now a luxury that hospitals cannot afford. Patients no longer are admitted to hospitals simply for testing unless their condition requires a specific hospital service, such as the administration of intravenous fluids. All insurance companies and third-party payers, including Medicare, now pressure doctors to get their recovering patients out of the hospital fast. Just being weak or exhausted is considered no reason to lie in bed doing "nothing" when your bed can be filled with a more acutely ill patient whose bill, in terms of reimbursement for care, tests, and treatment, can be compensating the hospital by an amount greater than what your current condition can generate. From this perspective, a "vacation" of this sort won't escape the attention of the hospital utilization reviewers.

More and more procedures are compressed into a shorter time span, with less time to recover between tests. In addition, the preparation for such tests may be debilitating. Enemas and the withholding of food before tests may lead to dehydration, which increases the risk of kidney damage; the danger increases with the injection of standard X-ray dyes. Repeated drawing of blood can sometimes lead to significant anemia. The overuse of laxatives can result in potassium loss. Waiting in the X-ray department for long periods is hardly a therapeutic procedure for sick people.

The result of such bureaucratic and cost-cutting policies is that those who are least able to tolerate the effects of testing are subjected to more tests within a shorter period. The potential for iatrogenesis multiplies.

Dealing with the issue of overtesting in the hospital can be tricky. If you do complain, or if you refuse to participate without getting an explanation, you delay the business of the hospital and you risk getting a reputation as a "bad patient." After all, would the doctor order a test that he or she didn't think was necessary at just the time it had been ordered? Checking is time-consuming, and time is a valuable commodity for hospital staff.

Your best defense against overtesting is to enlist allies, and the best ally you can have in the hospital is the nurse. The strategy here is for you to understand the reasons for tests and for you or your advocate to negotiate tactfully if you think there is a reason to avoid or postpone any of them.

Dealing with the Staff

Although the doctors write the orders, remember that hospitals are actually run by the nursing staff and other full-time personnel. For the most part, it's the nursing staff that bears the responsibility for the day-to-day care of patients and their well-being. There are nursing shortages in many hospitals, even in prestigious university medical centers. Unfortunately, once nurses have provided basic care, they may have little time left for other comforts and may often be delayed a long time in answering patients' calls for assistance. Having a family member or a private nurse or aide perform these duties may be either appreciated or resented by the regular nursing staff. On the one hand, the additional help may relieve the nurses of extra burdens, but on the other, it is a reminder to those personnel that they are unable to perform their jobs adequately. Your best assurance for a tolerable stay in a hospital is to develop a decent working relationship with your nurses. If you are able to accomplish this and make the nurses your allies, you are likely to have a far more comfortable time in the hospital than you will if you underestimate or neglect the importance of this relationship.

Many patients assume different personalities when they enter a hospital. Some become helpless and passive, following orders unquestioningly. Such patients regress to childhood dependence, permitting others to make decisions about their bodies and lives. Others become suspicious, hostile, and demanding. These patients are likely to end up receiving unfriendly, uncompassionate, or even ineffective care from nurses who put them at the bottom of their list of priorities. The suspicions and negative expectations of such patients frequently become self-fulfilling prophecies. Surely it might be difficult to stay sensitive to the feelings of your caregivers when you are ill and anxious about your own condition, but that sensitivity is precisely what's required here.

It's important to keep in mind that people who choose to go into nursing tend to see themselves as compassionate and helpful. Given a chance, that's how they're likely to behave. But nurses are neither your protectors nor your servants. If you treat them with respect and courtesy, you're likely to get courtesy and respect in return. As a token, you might start by addressing the nurses by name (nurses in most hospitals wear name plates) instead of as "Nurse."

Nurses operate in an environment of rules and regulations. Many of these rules are based on legitimate concerns for health or safety. Others may be arbitrary, capricious, and restrictive, and it's over the application of these rules that many of your negotiations will take place. The negotiations can address such issues as the times when your vital signs (temperature, blood pressure, pulse, and, sometimes, weight) are to be taken, the timing of your medication, and when your visitors may be allowed to come and when they must leave.

Nurses are frequently under pressure to get things done at certain times, even at the cost of a patient's convenience. For example, when doctors arrive in the morning, they expect to find the record of their patients' vital signs. As a result, nurses on the night shift normally record patients' temperature, pulse, and blood pressure before they leave. Nurses either may follow orders literally regarding the interval between medication, waking you just as you've fallen asleep or just before you were going to get up, or they may be more flexible. Regulations specifying visiting hours or the numbers of visitors allowed at one time, established to provide rest for patients, may be adhered to rigidly, without regard to circumstances, or stretched in order to accommodate visitors' schedules and patients' wishes.

In hospitals where regulations are rigorously enforced, you may have to appeal to the doctor to write orders to relax the schedules or to modify the visiting hours. If you want to avoid antagonizing the nurses, though, don't make it obvious that you're going over their heads. You might ask the nurse: "I understand your position, Ms. Robinson, but I'm very nervous about my operation tomorrow. Could you give permission for my wife [or husband or child] to stay an hour longer tonight, or do you need the doctor's permission?" While it isn't necessary to do so, it's always advisable to bring the nurses into any decision about waiving specific rules before you ask the doctor to modify them in the orders. This way you can keep the nurses as allies.

From time to time, despite your best efforts, you may not be able to establish rapport with one or more of your nurses. If a hostile relationship develops, you can ask for—and even demand—a different nurse. This is a fairly drastic measure that may involve a transfer to another room, and the news that you are a "bad" patient may precede you. However, it's important that your nurse—especially the daytime nurse, with whom you'll deal the most—be someone with whom you can get along.

Most complaints can be resolved by discussing them with the staff nurse with whom you have the most contact. Certainly this is true with minor complaints—long waits for your painkiller, for example, or problems with a technician who is rude. State your complaint clearly and calmly. If you get nowhere, talk with the head nurse on the floor. Normally, you'll have to go no further. If you do, ask to see the patient representative or ombudsman who is on the staff of an increasing number of hospitals. If you don't get satisfaction, at least you may learn the reasons for the problem.

If the problems are major—nurses who fail to answer calls regularly, who fail to notify the doctor of a change in your condition, or who bring the wrong medicine—the results may be serious. Notify your attending physician, who is ultimately responsible for your care. Keep in mind the negotiating rule: Focus on the problem and not on the people. There's a very practical reason for this caution. The doctor will spend more professional time with the nurses than he will with you, and he or she can't afford to antagonize the nursing staff.

If the problem still can't be resolved, the doctor may have you transferred to another section of the hospital, where a different nursing staff will care for you. The differences in nursing care in different parts of a hospital can be quite dramatic.

The Right of Refusal

Remember that you have a legal right to refuse any treatment, even in the hospital. You can say no to laxatives, X rays, excessive probing, medication, and any other procedure or treatment. However, few patients have the courage to refuse what they don't want, although many complain to doctors, nurses, and family. One study in 1983 counted only five refusals of any procedure in the course of one hundred days of patient treatment. Patients are vulnerable in the hospital, and they fear antagonizing doctors and nurses. Keep in mind that intelligent refusal may be a survival technique, especially if you think there has been a mistake in judgment or in execution.

Legal Issues

A body of law has evolved to provide protection for Americans so that they can make properly informed choices about their medical care and exercise some control over what happens to their bodies. Some of these protections are actually written into the laws of many states, some of them arise from precedents established by the courts, and some originate in common law as well as in the ancient ethics of medical care.

Informed Consent in Theory and Practice

During the first half of the twentieth century, the courts grappled with the principle of *disclosure*—the idea that a patient has the right to know what the doctor proposes to do to him or her, and the risks involved. While the principle of disclosure was widely affirmed, it was often disregarded in practice. If a patient submitted to a procedure, it was generally assumed that, unless the doctor fraudulently misrepresented the actual procedure, the patient was aware of what the doctor intended to do.

In the late 1950s, the courts began to ask whether, in addition to disclosure, patients are also entitled to *self-determination* — the decision about whether the proposed procedure is acceptable. What evolved was the doctrine of *informed consent*, charging the doctor with an affirmative duty to tell patients about the risks of the proposed course of action and *providing plausible alternatives*, with their accompanying risks and benefits.

The courts weren't prepared at the time to deal with such difficult questions as: Just how much are doctors required to disclose? Are they to disclose the risks and benefits of no treatment as well as of the treatment proposed? How many alternative treatments are doctors required to present—or even to know about? Instead, the courts retreated to the old principle of "professional standards of care," permitting doctors to disclose only as much as other doctors customarily disclosed. The ideal of patient self-determination in medical decision-making, proclaimed in the court opinions of the 1960s and 1970s, quickly evaporated in its application.

Many physicians believe that patients really don't want to know anything beyond the doctor's recommendations. However, a survey conducted for a 1982 report by the President's Commission for the Study of Ethical Problems in Medicine and Biomedical and Behavioral Research found that 96 percent of patients wanted to know everything about their conditions and upcoming procedures.

In practice, informed consent from the physician's standpoint is often a mere formality that allows patients to be told of the risks of the proposed treatment, after which they are expected to sign a form that will protect the doctor from litigation. In this view, informed consent is a form of defensive medicine that legitimizes the doctor's decision. To the patient, presented with a legal document that he or she had no hand in preparing and that lists the awful consequences of treatment gone awry, informed consent means either signing the document as it has been written or being refused medical treatment.

Such perceptions have little to do with the spirit of informed consent envisioned in judges' ringing declarations about the right of a patient to be "master of his own body" (*Natanson v. Kline*, 1960) and the right "to determine what shall be done with his own body" (*Canterbury v. Spence*, 1972).

The *spirit* of informed consent is the subject of much of this book. It suggests an ongoing process between doctor and patient that involves information-sharing and clear communication about diagnosis and treatment, about benefits and risks, and about alternatives and preferences. It implies a therapeutic alliance between doctor and patient.

If you are involved in this kind of relationship, signing the consent form merely affirms what you and your doctor have already clarified and decided. If you have questions about anything on the form, put the pen down and ask the doctor to clarify the matters that you don't understand or that concern you.

If your relationship does not involve this kind of therapeutic alliance, don't be rushed into signing the consent form. Don't lift the pen until you've read the agreement carefully. If there are sections in it that you don't understand or have doubts about, ask the doctor or request that someone from the hospital administrator's office clarify them for you. The fact that you are asked to sign the form should tell you two things: There is some risk involved, and both doctor and hospital are protecting themselves. Make sure you understand the risks before you sign. Reserve the right to write in stipulations. Be aware, though, that if the doctor or the hospital disagrees with your written comments, they may refuse to perform the procedure.

Page 129 shows the consent form for surgery that is used in a 700-bed hospital in Sarasota, Florida, where the authors live. It's typical of a reasonably well considered consent form that's not designed to trap or trick the patient. Yet, even in this form, no space is allotted for the patient to write in any reservations, conditions, or stipulations.

Note that clause 1 specifies the doctor who will perform the operation, "with such assistant(s) as he deems appropriate." If the form that you are asked to sign states, as many do, that the operation will be performed by this doctor "and/or such associates or assistants as he may select," you should be alerted to the possibility that the surgeon you expect to operate on you may delegate the task to someone else, as is quite common in a teaching hospital. If you are concerned about a possible substitution, clarify the question with the doctor and let him or her know that you want to cross out the first "or."

You should certainly ask the surgeon to clarify clause 4. As it stands, it provides blanket authority for the performance of procedures that you may or may not want performed, and it violates the spirit of informed consent. If you and the doctor have agreed that certain procedures are specifically not to be performed, ask if he or she has objections to your stipulation to that effect on the bottom or back of the form. If the doctor does object, you should certainly find out why.

SARASOTA MEMORIAL HOSPITAL, SARASOTA, FLORIDA   02-9020 R1/85

Name of Patient: _____

   1. I authorize performance in Sarasota Memorial Hospital of the following operation:

_____

Procedure or Treatment

by Dr. _____, as surgeon, or physician, and with such assistant(s) as he deems appropriate.

I consent to the performance of operations, procedures and treatment in addition to or different from that named above if, during the course of the operation, the above-named physician considers such addition or change necessary, appropriate, or advisable. I authorize the agents and employees of the Sarasota County Public Hospital Board to render such hospital care and services that are customary and necessary with respect to all such operations, procedures and treatments.

   2. I have conferred with the said physician and/or other physicians about the nature and purpose of the operation or procedure, the possibility that complications may arise or develop, risks which may be involved and possible alternate methods of treatment.

   3. I understand that no warranty or guarantee has been made as to the results or cure.

   4. I authorize and direct the above-named physician and/or his associates and assistants to provide such additional services as they deem reasonable and necessary including, but not limited to, the administration and maintenance of anesthesia, the administration of blood and blood products and the performance of services involving pathology and radiology.

   5. Any tissues or parts surgically removed may be retained or disposed of by Sarasota Memorial Hospital in accordance with its accustomed practice.

   6. I have received an explanation of this operation or procedure as stated above, and I give my informed consent to its performance. I hereby release Sarasota Memorial Hospital, its employees, agents and medical staff from any further responsibility of obtaining additional permission to perform this operation or procedure.

I have read this form carefully before signing it and have been given an opportunity to question my physician about this operation or procedure.

Witness (must be an adult) _____   Signature* _____

Date: _____ Time: _____

*Where the patient is incapable of signing and another person signs in his stead, complete the following:

State why the patient is not able to give consent personally (nor to sign this form).

Explanation:

___ Minor—any unmarried male or female who has not reached his/her 18th birthday.

___ Unconscious

___ Physical Condition

___ Other _____

Relationship of signer to patient: _____

If patient is a minor, name of parent or guardian: _____

Patient Identification

Clause 5, as it stands, could allow the destruction or discarding of surgically removed tissue that has not been adequately analyzed. In the event of a poor outcome, such an analysis could constitute important evidence. Talk with the doctor, and make sure that all tissue will be sent for pathologic examination. You can even ask the doctor to have copies of the pathology reports and the surgical report made for your file.

Informed refusal. A concept that is complementary to informed consent is the legal notion of *informed refusal*. This concept is not yet written into the civil statutes, but it has been clearly established in court cases.

Since it is *assumed* that if a doctor offers treatment, the treatment will be of some benefit, then refusing treatment presumably will in some way jeopardize the patient's health and well-being. Court cases have clearly established that patients must be informed of the consequences of their *refusing* a particular therapy or diagnostic procedure, so that they can make valid choices among all of their options.

A 1987 study at the University of Virginia showed that a patient's refusal was commonly based on mistakenly held beliefs, anxiety, fear, depression, and denial of the illness. In addition, in most of the cases the doctors readily accepted the patient's refusal, as if their recommendations had been offered on a take-it-or-leave-it basis. Unfortunately, many physicians simply don't take the time to explore the patient's reasons for the refusal, shrugging off their responsibility to inform the patient of the possible consequences. Such situations demonstrate a troubling lack of perception on the part of the doctor. The patient has the right to *informed* refusal. *Uninformed* refusal may be a sign of the physician's failure to communicate.

If you are reluctant to proceed with a diagnostic or treatment procedure, be frank and open with the doctor. Explain your reasons, even if you are afraid that they will be seen as silly or irrational. Very often the doctor will be able to correct misconceptions or allay your fears, allowing you to move ahead with the necessary care. But don't count on the doctor to probe for misconceptions without your first volunteering your feelings about the refusal.

Who can give consent? Court decisions and state laws are quite specific about *who* is in charge of making medical decisions. As long as you are mentally and physically competent to do so, no one but you may make your diagnostic or treatment decisions.

Illness, medications, or hospitalization can cause emotional distress and anxiety, and can reduce attention span, but none of these factors necessarily makes someone incompetent. Incompetence is a legal concept that refers to a determination that a person is generally unable to make decisions for himself or herself. An impairment of intellectual function may prevent someone from balancing a checkbook, but such impairment may not constitute incompetence in making health decisions. Unless a person is unable to cooperate with a medical evaluation, and evidence of general intellectual impairment is corroborated by substantial evidence from caregivers, the courts would almost certainly affirm that person's capacity to make medical decisions.

When decisions must be made for the patient. With few exceptions, the patient has the right and the opportunity to select the goals of therapy and to play a major role in accomplishing those ends. However, there are times when this isn't possible, either because a patient's condition demands that there be absolutely no delay or because the patient isn't capable of making a reasoned choice. For a life-threatening acute event, like a heart attack, an auto accident, or a critical case of pneumonia, the doctor is expected to act promptly on the patient's behalf, and even the laws requiring informed consent may be temporarily waived. Keep in mind that this special state lasts only until the emergency is over and the condition is stabilized. At that point, the usual right to make decisions is restored to the patient or to someone else, either a family member or a designated surrogate decision-maker. (See chapter 8.)

When patients are comatose, or when they're incapable of understanding the range and consequences of treatment choices because of mental retardation, senility, or incapacitating illness, the decisions must be made by others. In such cases, decisions will be guided by the patient's clearly stated prior wishes, or choices will be made by a duly designated decision-maker acting on the patient's behalf. This decision-maker may be a legal guardian or a family member who may also happen to be a legal guardian.

Minor children are a special case, because while they may hold strong preferences for one treatment choice or another, they may not be able to act without parental consent. Certainly in a life-threatening situation, physicians will initiate therapy before obtaining parental consent. Less urgent but still serious situations can delay treatment until consent is obtained. If you have minor children who will be away from home, send with them a signed (and preferably notarized) written permission allowing an emergency room physician to initiate treatment in the case of trauma or another urgent-care situation. If you will be traveling and the children will stay at home, leave such permission with a trusted friend or relative.

Medical Malpractice and Defensive Medicine

Any medical decision to *do* something or *not to do* something carries the possibility of a mistake in judgment. In addition, even when the procedure is appropriate, the performance may result in a poor outcome, for a variety of reasons, ranging from pure chance to a physician's incompetence. In recent years, an increasing number of cases with adverse outcomes have been challenged by lawsuits brought against physicians for malpractice.

In the past, a medical malpractice suit was an oddity. According to a historical survey of medical liability reported in *MD* in April 1987, a family doctor, an obstetrician, or a neurosurgeon practicing in Illinois in the 1950s could expect to pay an annual premium of $25 for malpractice insurance. J. B. Spence, one of the nation's best-known malpractice lawyers, says that for the first 10 years of his practice as an attorney in Miami, he never heard of a malpractice suit.

The often-cited "malpractice crisis" is a relatively recent phenomenon. A remarkable paucity of reliable information is on record about malpractice cases, because no objective nationwide tracking system exists to follow trends in litigation or in jury verdicts. Information provided by such obviously biased sources as medical societies, hospital associations, and lawyers' organizations is often contradictory.

Nevertheless, according to a report in *Internal Medicine News* in 1987, it's clear that the number of malpractice suits filed in the last two decades has mushroomed, and reliable data show a rapid growth in the size of the awards made to plaintiffs over the years. However, they also show that, despite the publicity surrounding a small number of malpractice suits in which a large amount has been awarded to the plaintiff, most awards are far more modest than the public believes, with a median payment, in 1984, of $18,000, according to a General Accounting Office report.

The fact that almost half of all malpractice suits have resulted in damage awards or in settlements is cited by lawyers as evidence that a good deal of incompetent medicine is being practiced. Physicians' groups, on the other hand, see the figures as evidence that jurors are not able to understand or judge the complexities of medical decision-making.

One provocative finding to emerge from the GAO study is that almost half of the physicians involved in malpractice suits examined had previous claims filed against them. While a minority of physicians account for most of the malpractice suits, the rates that *all* physicians pay for professional liability insurance have accelerated dramatically in the last two decades. In 1987, the General Accounting Office reported that between 1982 and 1984 the average annual amount that obstetricians and gynecologists had to pay for malpractice insurance rose 72 percent, from $10,900 to $18,800. For the low-risk specialty of pediatrics, the average annual premium increased 21 percent, from $2,900 in 1982 to $3,500 in 1984. Figures released by insurance companies and surveys of their members by medical organizations indicate that premiums have soared since the time of the GAO report, especially for high-risk specialties. Today, premiums of as much as $100,000 are no longer unusual for such high-risk specialties as neurosurgery and obstetrics.

According to the Association of Trial Lawyers of America, however, the soaring rates have not significantly increased the *proportion* of doctors' gross annual income spent on liability insurance, a claim that seems to be corroborated by the General Accounting Office report of 1987, which found that, despite high increases in insurance premiums, the *average* cost of malpractice insurance was a relatively modest proportion—about 9 percent—of the average doctor's expenses. This proportion may vary, however, from as little as 4 percent in lower-risk specialties to as much as 40 percent or more in the higher-risk areas of practice.

While there is disagreement within the medical profession about whether or not malpractice litigation has reached "crisis" proportions, the increase in insurance rates and the perception of a crisis clearly have had an impact on how doctors practice medicine.

What is malpractice? Medical malpractice was first defined in an 1898 case, and the definition has not been significantly changed since.

In that decision, the court asserted that a physician or surgeon who takes a case "impliedly represents that he possesses, and the law places upon him the duty of possession, that reasonable degree of learning and skill that is ordinarily possessed by physicians and surgeons in the locality where he practices." Although the locality rule is being replaced by the recognition that uniform national standards govern medical training and practice, the rule remains that a doctor is guilty of malpractice only if he or she veers significantly from accepted medical standards, with resultant injury or damage to the patient.

A malpractice suit is a civil, not a criminal, legal action. It is based on the claim that a doctor's negligence or failure to meet reasonable standards of medical care (defined by the medical community) resulted in an injury to the patient, for which the patient may recover damages. An adverse outcome *or* negligent behavior in itself doesn't prove, or even suggest, medical malpractice. A patient has a basis for a malpractice suit only if he or she suffers injury that resulted from negligent substandard medical care by the doctor or hospital.

Changes in medical practice. We noted earlier how greatly Americans have enlarged their expectations of medicine. Technical advances in medical science have created the illusion of certainty in medical diagnosis and miracles in medical treatment. These expectations have also increased costs, contributed to depersonalization, and fostered bitterness when the results have been less than was expected. Moreover, the recent trend to regard patients only as health-care consumers implies their right to an acceptable outcome as reasonable value for the high cost of medical care.

Partly as a result of such changes in attitude, increasing numbers of suits are being brought against physicians by patients who blame their doctors for misdiagnosis or for poor results following medical intervention. The basis for malpractice actions varies with the type of medical practice. Internists tend to be sued mainly for misdiagnosis of or failure to diagnose cancer and heart disease, and for failing to monitor patients' drug needs and subsequent hazards. Surgeons tend to be sued for improperly performed procedures. For the most part, as long as the doctor has followed "acceptable" practice, the physicians have prevailed in the courts.

Nevertheless, doctors have considerably more than money and time at stake when they are sued for medical malpractice. Physicians' egos and their professional self-images are inextricably intertwined. A physician who has been sued, whether for valid or for frivolous reasons, suffers a blow to his or her sense of competence and professional pride. The doctor is likely to react with a combination of humiliation, bitterness, and defensiveness.

The result has been a tragedy for both physician and patient. The malpractice crisis has added significantly to the cost burden of the patient, because, while doctors and hospitals may pay insurance premiums, ultimately it's the patient who pays. Utilizing data from the American Medical Association's Socioeconomic Monitoring System, several medical economists estimated that the costs of malpractice insurance accounted for about 15 percent of the increase in the total health bill of the American public between 1983 and 1984. Furthermore, the increased cost of such insurance accounted for more than half of the increase in physicians' fees and charges during that period. While these figures are considerably higher than those calculated by the federal General Accounting Office noted earlier, there is little doubt that the rising premiums for the most part are passed on to patients.

In addition, physicians increasingly have practiced what has come to be called *defensive medicine*, taking precautions to protect themselves against a possible charge that they failed to consider every contingency in a patient's diagnosis and treatment. The practice of defensive medicine not only adds considerably to the monetary costs of medical services, but it increases the health risks to patients who are overtested and overtreated as a result of the exaggerated precautions. Interview surveys of physicians indicate that those who have been sued subsequently order more diagnostic tests, refer more patients to specialists, and exclude more high-risk patients from their practices than their colleagues who have not been involved in litigation.

Ironically, some defensive measures may add to the patients' costs without reducing the doctors' vulnerability. An editorial in the *Journal of the American Medical Association* in 1987 pointed out that failure to diagnose has been a classic basis for negligence suits against physicians. The result has been the defensive use of additional tests. However, reviews of closed malpractice suits show that the original problem wasn't based on an insufficiency of tests; it was a failure to follow up test results. From this perspective, increasing the number of tests is more likely to exacerbate the problem than to relieve it.

In certain areas of practice, some physicians have stopped doing procedures that involve high malpractice premiums. For example, a 1988 survey of family practitioners indicates that 18 percent of them had curtailed their obstetrical practice as a result of the high cost or unavailability of liability insurance.

Recent rulings and verdicts indicate that the courts have been looking more critically at the role of patients in adverse outcomes. In one 1983 case, the judge instructed the jury that in a patient-physician relationship, "the physician has the duty to his patient to exercise reasonable care in forming his diagnosis and rendering treatment, while the patient has the duty to exercise reasonable care in providing the physician with accurate and complete information and following his instructions for further care or further diagnostic tests." The jury's findings were that the physician had done his duty but that the patient had not.

Because the malpractice issue affects both physicians and patients, it's obviously in the best interests of both to avoid a confrontation. The specter of malpractice will always be present when the physician makes judgments, largely because doctors can rarely be sure how a patient will react if something goes wrong. As long as the physician makes the decisions alone, he or she assumes all the risks and will tend to act defensively.

From your point of view as a patient, you must choose one of two basic approaches to decision-making. If you choose to allow the physician to make the decisions for you, as do so many patients, it's your responsibility to inform the physician of all relevant information and to understand and follow his or her instructions. Since the physician now has the full burden of responsibility, you can expect the probability of being overtested and overtreated.

If you choose to participate in decision-making, you must also exchange relevant information. In addition, you must understand and agree on the risks and benefits involved and share the responsibility for the results of the decision. Because you have entered into a common acknowledgment of clinical uncertainty and a shared understanding of the possible outcomes, and because the decisions are being made jointly, your doctor is likely to feel far less pressure to practice defensive medicine. You can make your position clear by saying something like, "I know you can't offer any guarantees. But I would like us to make decisions together, on the basis of what is reasonable to expect from each option."

LEAVING THE HOSPITAL

The Discharge Agenda

You should have an agenda even for your departure from the hospital. The purpose of this discharge agenda is to identify your diagnosis and prognosis, to get accurate information about what took place in the hospital, and to be sure you know what program you're supposed to follow once you return home.

Your doctor might talk with you at the time of your discharge and outline certain procedures to be observed once you are home. He or she might even write some prescriptions. Nevertheless, verbal instructions and information may not be sufficient, because patients who are being discharged from the hospital are often tired, weak, and confused. Perhaps you are floating on a cloud of euphoria at the prospect of returning home or are depressed and anxious at the thought of leaving the security of hospital care and attention when you are still feeling vulnerable. In any event, patients usually aren't in a proper state of mind to absorb verbal information, especially if it includes complex instructions.

It's best to ask the doctor to write down the pertinent information, assuming his or her handwriting is legible. Most hospitals have fill-in forms that make this process easier. If such a form isn't available from the hospital, use the sample on page 138 as a guide for preparing your own or for having your family prepare one.

Even if the hospital does provide such a form, you might want to ask for a copy of your hospital discharge summary, the one that the doctor dictates for the hospital record. Two reasons make this a wise practice. Especially in a large hospital, where resident physicians or interns transcribe information from the hospital record for the discharge summary, errors can be made — even an erroneous diagnosis. In addition, particularly if a number of doctors have been involved in your care, you may never have been informed of a diagnosis or other pertinent data because each doctor may have assumed that another gave you the information. The basic facts should be on the discharge summary.

DISCHARGE INSTRUCTION FORM

Diagnoses   1) _____

                 2) _____

                 3) _____

                 4) _____

Surgery and
Procedures

                 1) _____

                 2) _____

                 3) _____

Medication	*Dose*	*Times of administration*
1) _____	_____	_____
2) _____	_____	_____
3) _____	_____	_____
4) _____	_____	_____
5) _____	_____	_____

Possible adverse effects _____

_____

Activity restrictions _____

_____

Dietary restrictions _____

_____

Special instructions _____

_____

Follow-up with Dr. _____ Date _____ Dr. _____ Date _____

SUMMING IT ALL UP

The doctor's office provides the setting in which you are likely to have the greatest freedom of choice and the greatest scope for negotiation. The hospital is the most restrictive.

Nevertheless, even in the hospital it's possible to exercise some degree of control over what happens to you. In fact, the very complexity and rigidities of a hospital make it even more important for you to become involved in your own health care. The involved patient, or the advocate who represents her or him, can negotiate within the limitations of reasonableness by learning the chain of command, establishing lines of communication, and maintaining them with understanding for hospital routine and respect for the hospital's staff.

In addition to improving the amenities that can make hospital stays more comfortable, there is a more compelling reason for you or your advocate to become involved in your care at the hospital. Despite their rules and regulations, despite their general efficiency, hospital staffs make mistakes. If you know what is scheduled for you, from tests to medication or surgery, you will be able to monitor whatever happens to you and to determine whether procedures are being properly executed. And the best way to learn what is scheduled is to ask questions.

A body of law has developed to protect the patient in the lopsided communication that takes place between lay people and medical practitioners. Foremost is the principle of informed consent, which is based on the right of the patient to self-determination, but which rarely goes beyond the protection of his or her right to be informed of risks. The so-called malpractice crisis is, in some ways, evidence of the failure of the spirit of informed consent. The best protection for the patient is forming a therapeutic alliance with the physician, in which common understanding and respect provide some assurance against the practice of defensive medicine, which too often includes overtesting, overtreatment, and the risks that accompany each.

6

Making Decisions About Medical Tests

The next time you're in your doctor's office, it's possible that he or she will say to you, "Let's run a few tests." For you, those "few tests" can involve anything from the drawing of a small sample of blood right then and there to a complicated, expensive, and potentially dangerous procedure that must be performed in the hospital. If you're in a hospital, you almost certainly will be punctured, thumped, and X-rayed in a series of testing procedures, some of which, you will be reassured, are "routine," but others of which are not. How necessary are all these tests? Do you have reason to question taking them?

Medical testing is big business. Doctors can now choose from more than 1,500 separate medical tests, and more are being developed almost every week. As of 1982, annual laboratory costs totaled $11 billion, and Paul Mehl, director of technical programs for the American Hospital Association, estimated in 1985 that laboratory testing was costing Americans $20 billion a year, with $5 billion being spent for tests performed in physicians' office labs, $5 billion for tests processed in independent labs, and $10 billion for tests in hospital labs. If you are hospitalized, up to one-quarter of your hospital bill is likely to be for inpatient laboratory and radiology services.

Moreover, this kind of reliance on diagnostic tests is increasing at a remarkable rate; a 1984 study found that the number of laboratory tests had increased by 10 to 15 percent a year since the 1950s. One study showed that at least one test was included in 54 percent of all visits to internists, in 37 percent of visits to family practitioners, and in 31 percent of all visits to pediatricians.

The proliferation of laboratory testing can and does mean more accurate diagnoses. However, research shows that when expensive new equipment is purchased by hospitals, there is an immediate increase in the perceived need for its use. Testing may also mean enormous expense, sometimes for questionable purposes. And in certain circumstances, testing can be more dangerous for you than the illness it is designed to detect or monitor.

WHY DO DOCTORS ORDER TESTS?

Bear in mind that tests themselves don't diagnose. Tests provide information that can be used in diagnostic decision-making; they are tools that can be used in the process of diagnosis. They can also be employed for a variety of other purposes, and they are used differently for these purposes by different doctors. Your doctor may:

- want to *screen* for a disease or problem (for example, a mammogram may be a standard part of a physical examination for women over a certain age)
- want to *confirm* a tentative diagnosis that the doctor has made on the basis of his or her familiarity with your medical history and your symptoms
- want to *rule out* a possible problem or diagnostic possibility
- want to *investigate* or *validate* an "*abnormal*" or questionable result of a previous test
- want to *monitor* your progress and make *course corrections* during a treatment process
- believe that testing will provide *reassurance* for you by making you feel that the examination is thorough
- want to *evaluate* how well your body *functions* in a specific area or capacity as a preliminary step in preparing a plan of treatment
- be practicing *defensive medicine*, establishing evidence to prove that he or she is covering every possibility, remote as it might be, in case anything goes wrong later
- want *more information*, even if the test results are not likely to influence the course of treatment
- order tests because that is *standard operating procedure*

Many of today's tests provide information that couldn't have been obtained just a few years ago. Used properly, medical tests can quickly and most often accurately provide information that could not be supplied by clinical observation alone. On the other hand, most patients and many doctors have an unwarranted faith in the ability of medical tests to identify problems objectively and unambiguously during the process of diagnosis. Test results can convince you that your diagnosis is accurate and precise, building a confidence that may not always be justified, given the limitations of the tests themselves and of human judgment in interpreting the results. In short, the value of medical tests depends largely on the knowledge, competence, and integrity of the physician who orders and uses them.

DO YOU REALLY NEED ALL THOSE TESTS?

Physicians themselves don't always agree on the value of medical testing or on the frequency with which tests should be used. As in other aspects of practice, doctors are aggressive (sometimes impulsive) or conservative (sometimes overcautious) in terms of their readiness to order and use tests or procedures. One study by Drs. S. A. Schroeder, K. Kenders, J. K. Cooper, and their colleagues found that some physicians in the same specialty—internal medicine—used common laboratory tests 17 times more often than did others.

Aggressive doctors may use tests for a variety of reasons, ranging from personal belief in the value of testing to professional bias based on their specialties or training. Even the age of the physician may be a factor. Another study by Drs. J. M. Eisenberg and D. Nicklin in 1981 found that younger physicians tend to order far more tests than their older colleagues. In some cases, the lure of the new technologies alone may be too much for a doctor to resist. Other physicians may be concerned about the possibility of a lawsuit for malpractice and may routinely and extensively explore every conceivable factor in resolving a problem, real or potential, to ensure against a finding that they didn't check out all possibilities. To the aggressive physician, an unresolved problem represents either a challenge or a threat. The image that such physicians tend to project is that of the conscientious doctor who is thorough and persistent in diagnosis and will spare no effort in ferreting out possible causes.

Conservative doctors, on the other hand, often hesitate to order tests as a matter of course, preferring a more deliberate "wait-and-see" approach. These physicians may be more concerned with the negative aspects of testing: the ambiguity, the costs, the discomfort, and the possible risk of injury that may result from some procedures. Fundamentally, conservative doctors may be willing to live with a degree of uncertainty for a longer period than are aggressive physicians, as we noted earlier. They may operate on the proposition that time often clarifies the problem—and sometimes resolves it. The image of the conservative doctor is often that of the cautious, deliberate physician who tries to spare the patient the cost, discomfort, and risks of unnecessary tests.

The two types of doctors differ more quantitatively than qualitatively in their use of tests; they calculate costs and benefits with different yardsticks. To the aggressive doctor, his or her conservative colleague may be unscientific and even negligent in not aggressively seeking answers. To the conservative doctor, the aggressive physician may be reckless in the relentless search for a resolution, even at a cost that may be disproportionate to the possible benefit.

Writing in *Medical World News*, Dr. Thomas A. Preston, professor of medicine at the University of Washington in Seattle and chief of cardiology at Pacific Medical Center, described a classic confrontation between the two types of physicians.

Dr. Preston had been asked by a colleague to see an 81-year-old patient who had heart disease. The man was mentally alert but suffered from severe symptoms that Preston diagnosed as cardiomyopathy, a generalized weakness of the heart muscle. Preston suggested drug treatment but no further diagnostic testing.

The intern and resident physician on the case insisted on cardiac catheterization, a complex and potentially dangerous invasive procedure, to look for coronary artery disease (CAD). Preston pointed out that the patient's symptoms showed no indication of CAD, but the house staff persisted.

"We think he deserves cardiac catheterization," asserted a third-year resident.

"What, specifically, does the patient deserve?" Dr. Preston asked.

"This man deserves to know whether he's a candidate for coronary artery surgery," the resident answered.

Preston pointed out that cardiac catheterization can lead to complications such as stroke, heart attack, and kidney failure. Did the patient deserve these? A patient gets a tooth pulled, Preston noted, if the extraction will promote his or her health, not because the patient deserves the procedure. "Don't we have a greater obligation not to harm our patients than we do to help them?" Preston asked. He reflected on the first principle of the Hippocratic Oath: *Primum non nocere* (First, do no harm), pondering about what had happened to the *"primum"* before *"non nocere."*

For the most part, *both* kinds of doctors tend to make their decisions on the basis of what *they* perceive to be the patient's best interest, but all too frequently without consulting the patient or asking for the patient's judgment. Nevertheless, it is you, the patient, who will be undergoing the tests, bearing the risks and the side effects — and paying for them. As the consumer in this business, you might want to keep in mind that the decision to have more or fewer tests, or to have them sooner or later — *unless there is a medically compelling reason to act quickly* — is more likely to be a personal decision that has to do with your own tolerance for uncertainty than it is to be a technical medical one.

The accelerating use of tests, with the increased costs and the potential to harm (or even kill), has led the medical establishment, the federal government, and private insurance companies to question the need for the great quantity of testing that is being done. In 1987 the American College of Physicians and Blue Cross/Blue Shield, the country's largest private health insurer, jointly issued the first set of guidelines designed to set limits around the use of routine hospital testing, and the Federal Health Care Financing Administration, which runs the Medicare program, has proposed national legislation to identify doctors who order "too many" tests.

Unfortunately — and increasingly — doctors' decisions to order tests, particularly high-tech imaging procedures (see below), are also affected by the lure of financial reward. When the doctor who orders the test also has a significant investment in the testing equipment, either alone or in partnership with a group of physicians or with a hospital, his or her objectivity in assessing the patient's need for a test can be easily compromised. A 1989 government report found that one in eight physicians who treated a substantial number of Medicare patients was an investor in a laboratory, indicating the potential for self-interest as a motivation in testing referrals.

Recent changes in medical practice have helped enhance the opportunities for such profits from testing. Not many years ago, if you had a urinary problem, you would have gone to your primary-care physician, probably your family doctor. If the doctor thought it was necessary, he or she would have referred you to a urologist for special diagnostic studies. Your primary-care doctor would have been kept informed of the tests that the urologist administered as well as of the diagnostic decisions. Your family doctor acted as your health-care manager.

Nowadays, patients tend to be more knowledgeable, and you are likely to arrange a visit with a urologist, a dermatologist, or a cardiologist directly, rather than through referral from your family doctor. Or you may have seen the specialist in consultation on a certain problem, and decide now to continue with specialized care, either for that or another matter. In any event, the testing program of a physician who acts as both the primary caregiver and the doctor performing specialized procedures is no longer subject to scrutiny by a referring physician. Without such informal peer review, the specialist who may be tempted to overtest can easily rationalize this behavior as the conscientious practice of medicine using the latest procedures.

The entire realm of testing contains a vast gray area in which the results of many tests that can be ordered for you may be of marginal value or may even be completely useless. In many such cases, the additional information that is gathered, often at considerable expense, may be relevant to your medical problems, but it may not influence treatment decisions in one way or another. With all this in mind, before you undergo an expensive or possibly dangerous test, it is often helpful to ask the doctor:

- What will this test tell us?
- Will the result of this test pin down the diagnosis or let me know what to expect in the future?
- Will the result of this test change the decision to treat, or alter the type of treatment?

If you're not satisfied with the answers you get, let the doctor know that you have reservations and simply say, "Unless there's a compelling need to do it right away, I'd like to wait before I take that test."

If you have strong feelings yourself—aggressive or conservative—

verify that your views and your doctor's are compatible. Letting your doctor make the testing decisions alone means that you are willing to let a physician substitute his or her personal and philosophical views for your own.

TYPES OF TESTS

The method of testing is related to the risks to which you may be exposed—risks with which you have every right to be concerned. The information that can be obtained from the tests constitutes the technical data that the doctor may need for diagnosis or for planning a treatment program. You also should know something about this area because the kinds of information that can be derived address the question of whether the tests are needed in the first place.

There is no universally accepted classification system for medical tests. But one method is to categorize tests as *easy, participatory,* and *invasive,* in terms of how the data are acquired. The type of information obtained can be thought of as a *physiologic "snapshot,"* an *anatomic image,* or an *assessment of function.* Many tests actually provide several kinds of information at the same time.

Easy Tests

The easier tests are the ones with which you're most familiar. They may be taken when you're ill or when you have a routine examination. These tests aren't necessarily easy to perform, but they don't require your active participation, and they tend to be easy on your body.

Blackbox tests. Easy tests include the chemical analyses of a body fluid or excretion, such as blood, urine, sputum, or stool. Most of these tests are processed away from the patient, who is involved only to the degree that he or she provides the sample. We characterize such analytic procedures as "blackbox" tests, because many chemical analyses literally go into black boxes—computerized equipment that processes the sample rapidly and automatically. In some cases, the sample is simply fed into the equipment and a printout emerges. There are machines that actually scan a blood sample, counting the number of blood cells per cubic centimeter, and even calculate the proportion of red and white blood cells in the sample.

As in any computer printout, the results can be most impressive, conveying a sense of accuracy and precision. For each analysis, you may find a specific value assigned to your sample and a range of acceptable values that are considered "normal." However, the data still must be interpreted and applied to your unique situation, and the aura of precision masks several problems that are built into any testing program based on the notion of "normality," problems that are described later in this chapter.

University Medical Laboratories

PATIENT NAME:		ROOM #:	
AGE:		ACCESSION #:	C1770115
COLLECTED:		RECEIVED:	02/29/88
REPORTED:		PT. ID #:	
REQUESTING PHYS:			

TEST NAME	RESULTS OUT OF RANGE	RESULTS IN RANGE	REFERENCE RANGE	
CHEM 27,COR RISK,CBC				
CHEM PROFILE 27				
GLUCOSE		105	70-110	MG/DL
SODIUM		145	130-150	MEQ/L
POTASSIUM		4.9	3.5-5.9	MEQ/L
CHLORIDE		105	100-112	MEQ/L
CARBON DIOXIDE		32	21-36	MEQ/L
ANION GAP		13	3-15	MEQ/L
BUN		15	6-20	MG/DL
CREATININE	1.2 H		0.6-1.1	MG/DL
BUN/CREATININE RATIO		13	9.3-24.4	
CALCIUM		9.5	8.3-10.6	MG/DL
CALCIUM,IONIZED		4.2	3.8-4.8	MG/DL
PHOSPHORUS		3.4	2.4-4.5	MG/DL
PROTEIN,TOTAL		7.0	6.0-8.0	G/DL
ALBUMIN		4.4	3.4-5.0	G/DL
GLOBULIN		2.6	1.3-3.5	G/DL
A/G RATIO		1.7	1.3-2.8	
BILIRUBIN,TOTAL	1.6 H		0.0-1.0	MG/DL
	SPECIMEN ICTERIC			
BILIRUBIN,DIRECT		0.3	0.0-0.3	MG/DL
BILIRUBIN,INDIRECT	1.3 H		0.0-0.6	MG/DL
CHOLESTEROL		189	RISK CLASSIFICATIONS:	
			< 200 MG/DL	DESIRABLE
			200-239 MG/DL	BORDERLINE
			>= 240 MG/DL	HIGH
TRIGLYCERIDES		51	40-160	MG/DL
URIC ACID		5.0	3.4-7.0	MG/DL
IRON		98	59-158	MCG/DL
ALKALINE PHOSPHATASE		144	80-285	U/L
AST(SGOT)		22	5-37	U/L
ALT(SGPT)		15	4-40	U/L
LDH,TOTAL		166	118-242	U/L
LDL (DERIVED)		117		MG/DL

```
                 LDL-CHOLESTEROL
              RISK CLASSIFICATIONS
     < 130 MG/DL          DESIRABLE
   130-159 MG/DL          BORDERLINE HIGH
   160 MG/DL OR MORE      HIGH
```

RISK CLASSIFICATIONS ARE BASED ON THE NIH EXPERT PANEL REPORT FROM THE NATIONAL CHOLESTEROL EDUCATION PROGRAM. CLIN. CHEM. 34:193-201, 1988.

HDL CHOLESTEROL		62	45-75	MG/DL

REPORT CONTINUED ON NEXT FORM

2PT25

Imaging tests. Another group of easy tests includes imaging procedures, such as X rays, nuclear and sonar scans, and magnetic resonance imaging. These tests permit the physician to see what's going on inside the body without guessing, thumping, or bumping.

The example that's most familiar to you is undoubtedly the simple X-ray examination. Sound waves and radioactive emissions are also used to produce images that are based on the relative density of body tissues or the concentration of substances in certain parts of the body. In the case of X rays, the denser the tissue, the lighter the image. One persistent problem with traditional X-ray images is the virtual impossibility of distinguishing between objects of similar density, such as muscle, water, and blood. To increase contrast in the images, an agent such as barium, iodine dyes, or even air is injected into organs or body passages; the problem is that every additional procedure or introduction of a contrast medium increases the risk to the patient to some degree.

There are other techniques that produce cross-sectional images of objects, distinguishing between tissues of similar density. CAT-scans, or CT-scans, the terms used to identify *computerized axial tomography*, refer to some of the most sophisticated of the X-ray imaging techniques. CAT-scanning is done with a special X-ray machine that takes many pictures from different angles and then moves the patient forward little by little, so that the instrument focuses on a specific portion of the body with each series of images. The images themselves are processed by a powerful computer. The computer constructs a cross-sectional view of each of the levels, or "slices," which is produced by combining the clearest parts of each of the pictures.

The machinery involved in CAT-scanning is extremely expensive; a body scanner can cost about $750,000. In addition, the use of the computerized equipment and the large number of pictures that are often needed for cross-sections combine to make the use of CAT-scanning equipment very costly—and increase the amount of X-ray exposure to which the patient is subjected. CAT-scanning should be used only when other forms of X ray will not be adequate, although many physicians have a tendency to order marginally needed CAT-scans simply because the equipment is available and the resulting pictures look impressive.

One major advantage of CAT-scanning is its relative safety when compared with the more dangerous invasive techniques that involve the intrusion of instruments into the body and that are described below. As the technology improves, and as more efficient production methods develop, the cost of CAT-scanning may well decline to the point where its use becomes increasingly more routine, replacing or augmenting invasive techniques. It is already being used in place of such invasive studies as *angiography*, which involves the injection of dyes into the blood vessels of organs. While angiograms are still widely used in heart examinations and for identifying blockages or swellings in blood vessels elsewhere in the body, CAT and MRI scans have virtually replaced the use of angiographic studies in the examination of the brain (except for aneurysms), the liver, the pancreas, and most other organs.

The remarkable advances in high tech have also made possible a wide array of imaging techniques that don't use traditional X-radiation. One of these is nuclear imaging, making use of short-lived radioactive substances that zero in on the organ under study and light it up with temporary radioactivity. Because of the short-lived nature of such exposure, there is no danger of injury from long-lasting radioactivity.

Other methods are being used increasingly in the search for safer imaging procedures. One of these is ultrasound, which works much the way radar and sonar do. It relies on the timing and pattern of the echo from sound waves that are transmitted at extremely high frequencies. Ultrasonic imaging is painless and is completely safe because it doesn't use materials that are radioactive or chemically charged. As a result, it is used routinely for a variety of tests, including the search for stones in the gall bladder and the movement of heart valves. Because ultrasound is so safe, it is used for obtaining pictures of unborn babies within the uterus of pregnant women in order to help alert physicians to current or potential problems.

Among the newest of the imaging techniques is magnetic resonance imaging, or MRI. The equipment surrounds the patient with a magnetic field and then uses a computer to assemble cross-sectional images (much as the CAT-scan does), recording the electromagnetic waves that the body emits. The results are impressive; so are the costs. MRI units can cost well over a million dollars, and the bill for a single procedure and the image analysis can run between $500 and $1,000.

MRI is generally recognized as the best way to assess certain types of brain and spinal cord problems. However, because of the potentially large profit margins involved in the use of this costly procedure, the potential for abuse exists; some neurological clinics have been accused of overusing MRI or of using it inappropriately.

The images that emerge from these techniques require analysis and interpretation by skilled personnel. Any interpretation, of course, relies on subjective judgment and may involve a degree of ambiguity. Skilled observers may disagree not only on what they see, but on what the findings suggest. And when two observers agree, establishing what statisticians call *inter-observer reliability*, neither may be accurate. Studies suggest that there is often a good deal of variability in such interpretations. The obvious safeguard, of course, is the second opinion, or even a third opinion when the stakes riding on the interpretation are high. Your own attending physician should consult with the interpreters to establish a consensus, so that you're not faced with a frustrating clash of opinion that you're not in a position to resolve.

Function tests. A third group of easy tests measures the efficiency with which your organs and glands are operating. Such tests not only provide information about possible functional problems, but help give you and your doctor feedback on changes that are taking place during treatment. Many of these function tests are referred to as "passive," even though they measure constantly changing body functions, because they don't require your active participation in the testing process.

One of the simplest tests to administer, and a remarkably "easy" one for the patient to take, is also an effective way of monitoring the efficiency with which the blood is circulating within your body. "Blood pressure" measures the force of the blood against the arterial walls, and it is determined with a simple instrument—actually a combination of instruments—called a sphygmomanometer. An inflatable cuff is pumped up to shut off temporarily the flow of blood in the artery just above your elbow. As the air pressure in the cuff is reduced, the operator listens through a stethoscope for the beat that signals the maximum, or systolic, pressure in that artery. The disappearance of the beat indicates diastolic pressure between heartbeats. The two numbers are read from a calibrated gauge or a mercury column, although some of the newer devices show a digital number. Those numbers are recorded as systolic/diastolic.

TWENTY-THREE COMMON TESTS

Test	Useful for general screening	Cost	Who should have it?	How often?	Accuracy, reliability, special risks, and other considerations
FIVE "EASY" PHYSIOLOGIC TESTS					
Blood pressure	Yes	Low; often free screenings	Everyone, starting in teenage years	Yearly, or more to monitor Rx	Results vary with the time of day, emotions, and thickness of arms. Rx decision should be based on multiple determinations.
Glaucoma check (tonometry)	Yes	Low; often free screenings	Everyone over 55 years or with vision problems	Every 1-3 years or to monitor Rx	Hand-held instruments vary tremendously and require anesthetic on the eye.
Hearing test (audiology)	No	Low; often free screenings	As indicated by symptoms	As indicated by symptoms	Reliable as long as wax is not blocking the ear canal and no congestion exists.
Electrocardiogram (EKG or ECG)	No	Low	People with risk-factors or symptoms of heart disease	For initial assessment and as needed	Highly reproducible, but high rate of false positives in healthy people and false negatives in heart disease. Serial tracings important to see change.

TWENTY-THREE COMMON TESTS (continued)

Test	Useful for general screening	Cost	Who should have it?	How often?	Accuracy, reliability, special risks, and other considerations
Pulmonary functions (spirometry)	Yes	Low-mod.; often free screenings	People with breathing problems, cough, heavy smokers, or occupational risk	For initial assessment and to monitor Rx and disease	Reliable and reproducible, but depends on ability of person to make a maximal breathing effort.
THREE "EASY" TESTS OF URINE AND FECES					
Urinalysis	Yes	Low	Women, diabetics, hypertensive, urinary or prostate problems	As indicated by symptoms	Reliable for presence of protein, blood, and sugar. Varies with hydration status. If infection suspected, culture may be needed. Microscopic exam less reliable.

Urine pregnancy test	No	Low	Women of childbearing age who have signs of pregnancy	As indicated by symptoms	Requires concentrated specimen (first one of morning). False negatives early in pregnancy. May need blood test to verify. If negative, and signs persist, see doctor.
Stool occult blood	Yes	Low	Everyone over 40, or those with history of colon problems	Yearly after age 50 or as desired	Many false positives and false negatives. Negatives should not be used to rule out problem. Positives should be followed up.
SIX "EASY" TESTS ON BLOOD					
Complete blood count	Yes	Low	People who are ill, who have symptoms, or are on certain medications; women who are menstruating (to detect anemia)	As indicated by circumstances	Very reliable when done by machine. Office check of hematocrit (anemia) very reliable.

TWENTY-THREE COMMON TESTS (continued)

Test	Useful for general screening	Cost	Who should have it?	How often?	Accuracy, reliability, special risks, and other considerations
Blood cholesterol	Yes	Low	Everyone by age 25. If there is a family history, then child should be tested.	If normal, every five years. More often if not normal or on Rx	Laboratories vary widely. Screening may be done nonfasting, but definitive assessment is done fasting with lipid profile. Repeat checks if elevated.
Blood sugar	Yes	Low	People with family history of diabetes	As indicated by circumstances	Highly reliable. Should be done fasting, or 2 hours after meals. Can be done at home to monitor insulin therapy.
Blood (serum) potassium	No	Low	People who take diuretics	At least yearly if on diuretic	Reliable, but should be processed quickly after blood is drawn or deficiency may not be seen.
VDRL (syphilis)	Yes	Low	Sexually active nonmonogamous people; anyone with sexually transmitted disease (STD)	When signs of STDs occur, periodically as desired	False positives occur and should be followed with confirmatory test. Will stay positive for years after infection.

AIDS antibody (HIV)	No	Low-mod.	High-risk groups: gay and bisexual men, IV drug users, those persons with many transfusions in past, sex partners of above.	Initially, then frequency based on exposure to risk groups	Lab proficiency varies widely. In low-risk populations, positive test should be repeated because it may be falsely positive. Predictive value of negative test is very high.
TWO "EASY" GYNECOLOGIC TESTS					
Pap smear	Yes	Low-mod. or mod. (depending on cost of doctor's exam)	All sexually active women (Pap smear is an occasion for a woman to have a gyn exam which includes breast BP, STDs, etc.)	Yearly	Reliability of lab varies widely. Errors in sampling (inadequate specimen) can occur. False positives occur and should be repeated. Prior to exam, avoid douches or chemicals.
Chlamydia culture	No	Low-mod. or mod. (see preceding note)	Sexually active women who are nonmonogamous or whose partners are not monogamous	As indicated by circumstances	10 to 20 percent rate of false positives and false negatives. Retest possible if negative. Positives (and partners of positives) should be treated.

TWENTY-THREE COMMON TESTS (continued)

Test	Useful for general screening	Cost	Who should have it?	How often?	Accuracy, reliability, special risks, and other considerations
THREE "EASY" IMAGING TESTS					
Chest X-ray	Controversial	Low-mod.	May be of benefit in screening heavy smokers or those at occupational risk. Otherwise only in those with symptoms of lung or heart disease.	As indicated by symptoms. Yearly screening of heavy smokers may be helpful.	Problems arise with interpretation, which varies with skill and experience of the doctor. Clinical correlation is essential and comparison with old films is very important. X-ray exposure is minimal and is not a risk.
Mammogram	Yes	Mod.	Women over 40; younger if there is a positive family history of breast cancer	Ages 40–50, every 1–2 years (yearly if family history is positive), over 50, yearly	Using low-dose technology, risk of repeat exam is far less than benefit at any age (risk is very small). Comparison with prior exams is essential. Cancers can be detected early in subclinical state, but false positives occur. 10 to 20 percent false negatives mean that lumps must be biopsied even if mammogram is negative.

Bone density	No	Mod.-high	Women at high risk for osteoporosis	As indicated and not repeated	No risk, but value of this as a screen is low unless it markedly alters Rx strategy.

ONE PARTICIPATORY FUNCTION TEST

Exercise treadmill test (with thallium nuclear image)	No	High (Very high)	People with symptoms of heart disease or high-risk patients planning vigorous exercise program	As indicated by symptoms for diagnosis. Done to assess risk and functional recovery after heart attack.	Little risk but limited by effort and by exercise capability. Often false positive, especially in young men and in women of all ages. Not productive in healthy people without risk factors. Medication may limit predictive value of test.

TWO INVASIVE DIRECT-LOOK TESTS

Sigmoidoscopy (flexible)	Yes	Mod.-high	Everyone over 50; people with positive fecal occult blood, with colon symptoms, or with family history of such problems	Every 3–5 years after two consecutive negative tests	Little risk although perforation of colon can occur. Preparation (clean-out) is important. Totally dependent on skill and care of examiner. Short rigid scope reaches only 1/3 the length of flexible scope and is often very uncomfortable.

TWENTY-THREE COMMON TESTS (continued)

Test	Useful for general screening	Cost	Who should have it?	How often?	Accuracy, reliability, special risks, and other considerations
Colonoscopy	No	Very high	People with polyps, removal of colon cancer, persistent blood in stool, persistent colon symptoms	Depends on initial findings	Uncomfortable, often requiring injected sedatives. Extensive preparation of liquid diet and cleansing laxatives and enemas. Dependent on skill of specialist. Diagnosis and treatment often in same procedure.
ONE INVASIVE IMAGING TEST					
Cardiac catheterization and coronary angiogram	No	Very high	People with serious heart disease who may benefit from by-pass surgery, valve replacement, or other surgery, or angioplasty	As indicated by need for intervention	Very small risk of death in experienced hands, but irregular rhythms can occur that require prompt reaction. Requires hospital stay and immobility afterward to prevent bleeding complications. Totally dependent on specialist's skill for test performance and analysis. Dye reactions can occur.

There is general consensus in the United States that readings higher than 140/90, taken while the patient is resting, may be a warning of hypertension, or high blood pressure. Because blood pressure is subject to many influences, your doctor should be reluctant to accept any one reading as "true." He or she may make repeated measurements during one visit and will probably repeat the test over the course of several visits. The doctor may ask you to take periodic readings at home with a low-cost home device before starting you on medication.

Another familiar functional test is the *electrocardiogram*, usually referred to as ECG or EKG, which constitutes a record of changes in electrical potentials that occur in the heart under a variety of conditions. The ECG may be administered either as a passive test or as a participatory one (see below).

A large number of the function tests measure the response of the body's glands to a stimulus. These glands operate much the way a thermostat does; they will "turn on" to secrete hormones when the blood level of these hormones falls below a certain point. By administering substances that control the gland production, the physician can "fool" the gland into turning on or off, to see if it is functioning properly.

Often the level of a hormone can be measured directly in the blood, and this is useful in assessing the functional status of an endocrine gland. The adrenal gland produces cortisol, which controls the way in which the body reacts to infections or other illness. Cosyntropin, which is chemically identical to a portion of the body's own adrenal-gland-stimulating hormone ACTH, can be injected to activate the gland. If the adrenal gland is working properly, the cortisol level in the blood should double within 30 minutes. The response to the cosyntropin is an easy way to determine whether the gland is functioning properly, and this test can help differentiate between primary and secondary failure of cortisol secretion.

Such function tests are usually administered in the medical laboratory. A simple function test like the adrenal-gland-stimulation test may cost close to $100. A thallium exercise stress test, which combines electrocardiographic monitoring, treadmill exercise, and nuclear imaging, can cost $1,000 or more. Be aware that the interpretation of all the function tests, passive or participatory, requires a good deal of caution. For example, the level of plasma cortisol or even blood sugar, as is true of any hormone or hormone-controlled compound, is intimately related to time of day. Sugar level, in particular, is also affected by the nature and the times of meals. As with so many other tests, patterns of change may be far more important than "snapshots" of status. Moreover, a number of tests administered at intervals may help to minimize the variations that emerge from the subjective interpretations of results.

Participatory Tests

Mention has already been made of exercise stress tests, which require the active participation of the person being tested. This test involves your mounting a treadmill, the speed and incline of which are adjusted so that your ECG can be recorded under changing levels of physical activity. Sometimes the test is combined with imaging studies that use nuclear tracers such as thallium, which are injected at the peak of exercise in order to determine the adequacy of blood flow to the working heart muscle. Another common participatory test is the pulmonary function (breathing) assessment. It measures how well you can breathe in and out, and the result can indicate if there is an obstruction to the airflow.

Participatory tests require voluntary effort. Moreover, the accuracy of the results depends in large part on the effort you expend. For example, the exercise stress test and the pulmonary function test assess the extent of either circulatory or breathing reserve. The results may suggest to the doctor that your functioning may be limited by organ damage or disease, and they may be an indication of whether you have the reserve capacity to endure further stress, such as surgery. If your efforts were halfhearted, the doctor may misinterpret your lack of effort as poor functioning. Because the accuracy of the measurements rests so heavily on your own effort and involvement, these tests are truly participatory.

Invasive Tests

By far the most complicated tests are those that are referred to as "invasive." These tests involve intrusion into your body, either in the process of obtaining a sample of tissue or in getting an image that cannot be obtained from outside the body. Many of the invasive tests use combinations of other techniques; some X-ray procedures, chemical analyses, and function tests are invasive. Any test in which the body is entered by something larger than a small, short needle is potentially painful or dangerous and can be justified only if the results cannot be obtained in simpler ways. Even puncture by a needle can be dangerous, especially if it extends deep into the tissues, possibly causing bleeding or damage to an internal organ.

Obtaining a clear image of an organ or a blood vessel with external X rays is sometimes difficult to do. To heighten the contrast and sharpen the image, agents such as iodine dyes often are injected into the body, sometimes by direct injection with a needle. Dye can be inserted into a joint for an arthrogram, into the spinal canal for a myelogram, or even directly through the abdominal wall into the bile ducts for a cholangiogram.

Sometimes X-ray contrast materials must be injected into deep internal organs that can be reached only by using long catheters. These are narrow hollow tubes that are inserted into blood vessels in order to deliver the dye to the heart or other organ, or to the blood vessels themselves. The resulting picture of the blood vessels is referred to as an angiogram, and the procedure by which the catheter is passed into the heart to inject dye or measure pressures is called a *cardiac catheterization.*

The use of such catheters always presents a degree of risk; there is the possibility that as it travels through a blood vessel, a catheter will dislodge cholesterol plaques that may eventually block an artery downstream. Catheters also can irritate the heart during catheterization, causing abnormal rhythms which can be life-threatening if not treated promptly. Furthermore, injecting dyes into blood vessels in the head carries the risk of stroke damage. Because of the risks, angiography and catheterization are not procedures to be undertaken casually, and they must always be performed by a highly experienced and competent specialist. In most hospitals, only certified specialists are permitted to perform arterial catheterizations.

When X-ray studies aren't sufficient to examine organs properly, scoping techniques are often employed. Rigid, or semirigid, hollow tubes are inserted through a body opening. These are illuminated at one end and contain an eyepiece at the other, so that the examiner can look directly into a lung, the colon, the esophagus, or other interior parts of the body, and even photograph what is seen. In addition to looking into natural body orifices, the examiner may make a small hole in order to insert a scope into the abdominal cavity to examine the ovaries or other structures (laparoscopy), or into a joint such as a knee to look at the internal structures (arthroscopy).

Rigid scoping, of course, has some built-in limitations. For one thing, rigid scopes can't be bent around corners. The problem has been solved with the development of fiber optic technology. Bundles of long, flexible glass filaments can be bent to follow virtually any contour. Each of the light-sensitive glass filaments passes back light, so that the entire bundle will create a picture that is made up of microscopic dots, something like the picture on your television screen or in your daily newspaper. Because of the flexibility of this scoping technique, an experienced interpreter can use it to search for tumors throughout the lung, as in a bronchoscopy, or to survey the entire length of the colon, as in a colonoscopy.

Flexible and rigid scopes can also provide access to otherwise remote areas of the body so that dyes can be introduced to facilitate X-ray imaging in the bile ducts or in the tubes leading from the ovaries to the uterus. In addition, a skillful examiner can pass special probes and forceps (grasping instruments) into otherwise inaccessible areas of the body to obtain samples to examine microscopically. Specialists also can use scopes to perform corrective or surgical procedures, such as stopping a stomach ulcer from bleeding, removing a torn cartilage from a joint, and even "tying the tubes" of a woman for permanent birth control.

The risks and benefits of invasive tests. As we've discussed, the risks of invasive testing can be high. If a needle is pushed through the skin to get a sliver of tissue from the liver or another organ, there is always the possibility of bleeding or organ damage. While it's usually safe to look into either end of the intestinal tract, the possibility exists that the esophagus or the colon can be ruptured (perforated) in the course of the examination, especially if disease or inflammation is present.

On the other hand, often both the risks and the expense of such procedures are clearly warranted, because vital information may not be available by using other alternatives. Sometimes the invasive techniques simply may be preferable to the alternative procedures; in many cases, they can replace the major surgeries that were necessary in the past to remove polyps and stop bleeding in the intestinal tract, to repair torn cartilage in the knee, and even to open up blocked blood vessels in the heart. Often they can constitute test and treatment simultaneously (see chapter 7).

As invasive procedures increase in complexity, the dexterity and observational skill of the person performing these procedures will become more and more important. Unlike the blackbox testing, which often produces an objective analysis of a sample, the manipulation of a scope or catheter and the proper recognition of what is seen during the testing procedure are the factors that make the accuracy of many invasive tests more a function of the skill of the physician than a function of the test procedure itself.

The decision to proceed with an invasive test is a judgment that should be made by you and your doctor together only after you have discussed the benefits and risks, the expenses and the alternatives. Remember that many invasive tests can involve costs and risks that rival those of surgery. Like surgery, however, invasive procedures can sometimes offer benefits that aren't available through the use of other procedures. Before you agree to submit to an invasive test, you should be convinced that these benefits are worth the costs and risks of the procedure.

INTERPRETING TEST RESULTS

The faith that most Americans have in the accuracy of test results may not be entirely warranted, as we noted earlier. The aura of scientific authority conveyed by the sophisticated procedures and the apparent precision of the results of modern biomedical testing tend to disguise some persistent problems.

Many test results provide only measurements—raw data that must be interpreted. One persistent problem is the confusion of raw data, such as an ECG printout or an X ray, with the conclusion that a doctor may draw from it. When a doctor says, "Your ECG shows a heart attack," he or she really means, "On the basis of the information that is present in the ECG, together with what I know about you, I believe that you've had a heart attack."

Often, the results of a study at any particular moment are less important than the changes or trends that can be observed, either during the test itself or from one test performance to another. *Because you are different from anybody else on earth, the changes that take place in your readings are far more significant than are your deviations from the norm.* Here are some reasons for approaching test measurements with caution.

Any single test result can be like a snapshot. It may show where you are at that moment, but it doesn't show how you got there, or where you're going. We have observed how remarkably body functions vary with time of day, diet, emotional state, and a multiplicity of other conditions, so a single snapshot may not show the "real" you, or it may show you in a distorted pose. More important, such a snapshot doesn't indicate patterns of change. Because of these variables, tests must often be repeated or results must be compared with previous test results so that patterns may emerge.

Since no two individuals are exactly the same, your blackbox print-out may show that a function or the composition of your blood is within the "normal" range—but for *you*, the value may be abnormal. Similarly, it may show an abnormality that doesn't really exist, because the value may be normal—for you. Some individuals will consistently record measurements that appear to be abnormal when, in fact, they have no real problem.

Test results may be misleading without additional data. For example, a blood count may show an unusually high level of hemoglobin. Is this good or bad? The number itself tells little; if you're a heavy smoker, your doctor may explain that you are adapting to the smoke "smothering" your red blood cells. On the other hand, if you don't smoke, your doctor may be concerned that something is wrong with the blood production itself.

To minimize these and similar problems of interpretation, all physicians should—and many physicians do—refer not only to your medical history, but to previous test results, to ascertain if there have been significant changes. Your doctor may prefer to analyze the raw data personally, rather than rely solely on the interpretations of other doctors, such as radiologists or pathologists, who aren't likely to have any information on your personal or family medical history.

It has been estimated that for some body functions, such as the level of cholesterol in the blood, up to three repeat samples may be required to identify an individual's base-rate profile. This underscores the importance of having access to your medical records so that your previous readings are readily available. One way of establishing some continuity to your medical records is to maintain a continuing relationship, whenever possible, with one doctor who keeps track of your test results. If this isn't possible or feasible, or if you change doctors, or if you travel a good deal, you should consider keeping your own file of medical reports and summaries to show to your doctors.

HOW ACCURATE ARE MEDICAL TESTS?

Patients often view tests as a way of ascertaining with certainty whether or not they have a disease. In fact, many patients assume that tests are scientific and objective, and that the newer a test is, the more information and the better the answer it provides. As a result, many doctors report that they frequently order tests because their patients seem to need the assurance of certainty—or the illusion of certainty. Physicians themselves are usually far more aware of the limitations of testing.

The accuracy of a test is determined by a number of factors, including: the degree to which the test measures accurately what it is supposed to measure; the accuracy with which the measurement is made or with which the test is interpreted; and the nature of the patient.

The first factor, known as *test validity*, is one over which you're not likely to exercise much control, because it's largely a technical question, the answer to which emerges from experiments, studies, and, ultimately, from the cumulative experiences of the medical community. The question of validity becomes a problem when a test is found to be less accurate in identifying problems than is generally considered reasonable in diagnosis. Invalid tests don't usually remain in use very long after they are discredited.

If you concern yourself at all about the accuracy of tests, you're likely to be most concerned about the second factor. You may wonder about the possibilities of errors in laboratory measurement and in the interpretation of test results. You're more likely to think about the issue if the doctor tells you that the test results are *positive*, meaning that they indicate that a problem exists, than if he or she tells you that the results are *negative*.

Major problems, however, may result more frequently from false negative results, rather than from false positives. False positives often have a built-in correction mechanism. When physicians get a lab report suggesting the presence of a disease or a problem, they are likely to order another test or to repeat the test to verify the lab report. On the other hand, if the physician gets a negative report, he or she is probably going to tell you that there is no problem. At this point, you are likely, in your relief, to stop thinking about the matter and to ignore the symptoms that may have brought you to the doctor's office.

While there is a possibility of error in any test, mistakes are more likely to occur in some kinds of tests than in others. Certain tests, like those for cancer, pregnancy, or AIDS, provide answers that are binary—they are either "yes" or "no." Others, like those for ulcer, diabetes, anemia, or coronary artery disease, provide information on a continuum of degrees of severity; they tell you *how much* or *how bad* a condition may be.

One major difference between these tests is that the yes-no answers usually are provided directly by test results. On the other hand, the tests that measure where your problem may lie on a scale must usually be interpreted, and every additional step in testing introduces another place where an error can occur. Because of this, aside from the mistakes that can occur in the administration or the laboratory handling of the test, you must also be concerned with the variations in the ways in which different observers interpret the test results.

If a major decision, such as whether or not to have an operation, rides on the accuracy of an interpretation of the test results, you might ask the doctor to have the test results (the raw data) sent to another specialist—a radiologist or a pathologist, for example—to verify the interpretation.

You must also be aware that despite close attention to safeguards, the possibility of error lurks in the performance of even the simplest yes-or-no test and in the information it yields. Errors in test results can and do occur for a variety of reasons: A machine may lose its calibration; testing chemicals may age and lose their potency; workers may be overworked and become careless; there may even be a mix-up of specimens.

Major laboratories have taken steps to minimize error. Some test chemicals and monitor calibrations daily, or they may use "master" specimens whose values are known in order to check equipment and procedures. Nevertheless, in the absence of regulatory oversight, errors occur in the best of laboratories. Even in states in which laboratories are supervised—only about half the states—mistakes happen.

However, the vast bulk of the millions of tests processed each year are handled quickly and competently in medical laboratories, a reality that leads many to think of lab work as infallible—a dangerous assumption, according to critics, who contend that human error is inherent in the testing process.

To many critics, a troublesome development is the dramatic increase in the number of tests administered and processed in doctors' offices. A major reason for this trend is the movement of care from more expensive inpatient settings to less expensive outpatient locations. While Blue Cross and Blue Shield noted a decrease of nearly 8 percent in hospital admissions between 1984 and 1985, this was matched by an almost equal increase in nonhospital physician visits. The current requirements of insurance companies to approve all hospitalizations before admission and the increased postdischarge review of the appropriateness of hospital services by almost all insurance providers further reinforce the trend.

While you can't protect yourself completely against the possibility of lab test errors, there are some precautions you can take to minimize the odds that the results will be distorted.

One source of testing error is based on the fact that "normal" readings are based on standard conditions: Such conditions may have to do with how you have to prepare for some tests. Among the questions to ask when your doctor orders tests are:

- Is there a particular time of day I should arrange to take this test?
- Should I eat my regular meal before I take the test? Are there any foods I should avoid?
- Can I drink liquids before the test?
- Should I continue to take my medication at the usual time?

In addition, you can take some precautions in guarding against some of the consequences of lab errors.

If the results of any test you take are positive, here are some of the questions that you might ask the doctor:

- What does this result mean?
- Is there something else we have to do now to verify this result? Does it pay to repeat the test? Or do we wait and monitor symptoms? How long should I wait, and when should I report back to you?

If the results are negative, you should ask for follow-up instructions:

- How long should I wait before contacting you if the symptoms persist?
- What other symptoms or signs should I be alert for?
- What other follow-up procedures should I take?

SCREENING TESTS: HOW USEFUL ARE THEY?

When you go for a checkup, you're likely to be given one or more "screening tests." These are tests that are used, more or less routinely, to check out the presence of a problem that may be common for a person in your age or risk category.

How useful are such screening tests? Advice from the medical establishment is contradictory. The American Heart Association and the American Cancer Society insist that regular checkups are the most effective way of detecting problems early enough to cure them. On the other hand, many experts scoff at mass screenings, contending that the level of successful disease detection in the general population is too low to justify the high costs of mass screenings in time and money.

Both sides are right. The key to the effectiveness of screening tests is an accurate assessment of the *base rate* (see chapter 3). Perhaps the most dramatic illustration of the role of base rate in accurate assessments emerges from the controversy raging in medical journals over screenings for AIDS.

In 1988 the Centers for Disease Control raised questions about the accuracy and precision of the standard tests for AIDS. The first screening is a blood test known as the ELISA test, which rarely misses an infected sample. The problem is that about 10 percent of the positive readings are in error; they indicate that a problem or a condition exists when, in fact, it doesn't. Fortunately, there is a second test that is administered in the case of positive results. The problem here is that this test, the Western blot test, gives false negatives in 10 percent of those with the infection and false positives in 5 percent of those who test positive. Moreover, the CDC points out, these false readings occurred in the best labs in the country, under optimum conditions.

However, the proportion of false readings depends far more on other factors, particularly the base rate, the risk level in the population that is being tested. In some ways, this may be the most important single factor that affects the accuracy of any test in diagnosing your problem.

The problems associated with base rates and Bayes' Theorem (see page 49) are aggravated in mass screening programs. When the Illinois state legislature mandated premarital AIDS screenings, they ignored the issue of base rate. While the tests that are used are quite reliable when applied to high-risk populations, the accuracy drops remarkably in a low-risk population, where the base rates are different. One report in the *Journal of the American Medical Association* calculated that a national compulsory premarital testing program would test 3.5 million people a year at an annual cost of well over $100 million. Of these, 1,200 infected persons would be identified, but as many as 380 people with confirmed positive results would be told incorrectly that they were infected—and more than 100 infected individuals would be told, incorrectly, that they were not infected. Dr. Renslow Sherer, of the Cook County Hospital and Clinic in Chicago, pointed out in the same journal that "despite . . . a positive predictive value of a positive ELISA of less than 30% in the general population, some physicians inform patients of ELISA results pending confirmatory tests."

Illinois abandoned mandatory premarital AIDS testing in 1989 because it turned out to be ineffective and far more costly than had been estimated.

The conclusion that emerges from reports in professional journals is that many physicians don't calculate base rates accurately when they deal with low-risk general populations. In government-mandated programs, such as those to screen for AIDS or for drug use, base rates aren't considered at all—and the chance of error in test results multiplies.

If you have been tested in a mass screening and are notified that your results are positive, and if you are truly in a low-risk group, you should certainly demand that you be retested.

Getting Involved in Screening Test Decisions

Many medical tests, especially those we have designated "easy," are routine and can yield a good deal of information. Nevertheless, there are risks and problems attached to certain kinds of tests, both easy and invasive, and one of the problems associated with the use of the easy tests, strangely enough, is that some are *too* easy. In an attempt to use screening tests that are safe, physicians often turn to techniques that are painless, inexpensive, and risk-free. The problem with this is that they may yield information that is questionable or possibly even useless. Some experts go so far as to doubt the value of many of those tests that are among the most widely used in screening.

Certain tests are very useful for screening when they are administered to "targeted" high-risk populations. They include tests for AIDS among groups with high-risk behaviors; tests for fecal occult blood for those at risk for cancer; and sigmoidoscopies, or scoping examinations of the lower colon, for those who have symptoms that may suggest a problem.

Many of these tests, on the other hand, are of limited value for use in general, or low-risk, populations, and they may even create traumatic new problems. The chance of error increases dramatically when such tests are used routinely to screen general populations. Nevertheless, studies reported in the *Morbidity and Mortality Weekly Reports* have shown that large numbers of physicians order AIDS testing of hospital patients, even in the absence of risk factors. Moreover, many of these patients are not even informed of the nature of the tests that are being conducted.

Consider the circumstances under which such tests for AIDS are often administered, especially in the hospital. When the technician comes to draw a blood sample, even if you are wary enough to ask what the test is for, you are likely to be told that it was ordered by the doctor—an ambiguous answer that most patients accept without question. Consider also the dire consequences of a positive result—including the false positives that become increasingly likely in a mass screening in a low-risk population.

As of this writing, in Minnesota, positive results of AIDS tests are reported not only to insurance companies, but to the state health department, so the consequences of false positive results can be devastating.

Just as the probability of false positives increases with inappropriate mass testing in a low-risk, untargeted population, so does the probability of false negatives. The wisest perspective you can take is to recognize the possibility of such false negatives in a mass screening program and to be alert to any symptoms that may develop.

In light of the widespread use of screening tests, you should be aware that you can take some precautions against inappropriate or improper testing procedures.

Some basic questions you should ask about screening:

• What can we learn from this test?

Be sure you understand the answer. For example, if you are told that the test is for HIV antibodies, you may not realize that this is one of the screening tests for AIDS. Keep asking until you get an answer you understand.

• Are there any reasons for you to suspect that I'm in a high-risk category for such a problem?
• Who will get the test results?
• What is the next step if the result is positive?
• What is the next step if the result is negative?

TESTING IN THE HOSPITAL

When you're confined in a hospital, your role as a patient is very different from your role as an outpatient in the doctor's office. Moreover, your testing program may differ greatly from the one you were accustomed to as an ambulatory patient.

Fragmented Medical Records

One of the first things that will happen to you when you are admitted to a hospital is that you will undergo a series of tests. Many of them may be repetitions of tests that you have already had, even in the past few days. There are two major reasons for such duplications.

Especially if you are confined in a large hospital, you may very well be receiving treatment from a group of doctors that you have never seen. More important, they have never seen you. They probably know little or nothing about you on a personal level, and if your medical and testing records are not readily available—if they have not been trans-ferred, or if they are "lost" somewhere in the bureaucracy of a large referral institution—these doctors will routinely order new tests. This persistent information gap is one of the reasons it's so important to have a personal link between the doctors inside the hospital and those you've seen outside.

Even if your records have survived and have reached the hospital doctors, staff doctors may not trust any data from outside their own institution. This distrust is especially characteristic of teaching hospi-tals, where residents and interns often refer to those who are not on the hospital staff as "LMDs" (local medical doctors) or as "outside physi-cians," whose decisions often are considered questionable.

Even when your own attending physician is nominally in charge of your case, the house staff is likely to be handling your day-to-day care and writing the orders. The best ways of assuring some continuity in your testing program in the hospital is to make some prior arrange-ments with your own doctor and to ascertain what will happen to your records after admission. Some basic questions:

- Who will be in charge of my case in the hospital?
- If it isn't you, will you be in direct contact with that person?
- Will you give me my medical records (or copies) to carry with me?

Hand-carrying your records and delivering them personally to the physician in charge of your case is probably the most reliable way of bypassing the black hole into which patients' records seem to disap-pear in most large hospitals. If your doctor is reluctant to give you the records personally, ask him or her:

- How will my records get to the hospital? What is the name of the person who will be receiving them?

At least you will know whom to ask once you're in the hospital. The black hole often works both ways. Once you're admitted, you should ask:

• Who will be sending reports to my doctor?

There may be times when you can anticipate a significant lag in the transmittal of your test reports. In such cases, you might also ask:

• Could you please give me copies of any important reports, or write a brief summary of my diagnosis and medications that I can take with me?

This last precaution is particularly important if you are treated away from home—at a referral center or while you're on a trip or on vacation.

IS HOME TESTING FOR YOU?

If the notion of performing your own medical tests at home surprises you, you may not have considered that you've engaged in medical testing every time you've taken your temperature. With the remarkable growth of the high-tech field, the home monitoring of body function has become very big business indeed. The American Pharmaceutical Association has estimated that the market for home test devices may be expected to reach $2 billion by the early 1990s.

This rapid growth is attributable only in part to the remarkable advances in the technology of lab testing devices—known in the field as IVDs, or in-vitro devices—that are suitable for use by lay people. Parallel with the technological advances has been the growth of the notion of autonomy, or patient self-determination.

Pharmacies, department stores, and discount outlets now stock devices and kits that range from sphygmomanometers for monitoring blood pressure, and otoscopes for ear examinations, to pregnancy kits, blood sugar monitors, kits to check for fecal (stool) blood, and even—in some outlets—kits for AIDS testing, all designed for self-assessment.

Some of these products are used for screening, to ascertain whether you have a certain condition or problem; these include the tests for pregnancy, for stool occult blood, and for AIDS, and they are usually single-encounter procedures.

Others are for monitoring your condition when you know you have a disease or even the tendency toward a disease. Included in this category of tests that are used periodically are those for blood pressure and for blood sugar.

Medical practitioners are divided over the value of such do-it-yourself devices. Some of the more conservative fear that patients simply don't know enough to interpret readings properly and thus are vulnerable to becoming overly alarmed, ignoring real danger signals, or sinking into complacency, depending on how they perceive the results. If even trained professionals often make mistakes, should patients be permitted to play doctor? Other physicians dismiss such concerns as remnants of the outmoded concept of "doctor-as-God." Proponents of home monitoring cite evidence indicating that diabetics who have been properly instructed in the use of home blood sugar tests tend to achieve far better control of their disease than do those who don't engage in home testing.

There is a major difference between single-encounter tests that indicate whether you have or don't have a condition and the repetitive tests that are used for monitoring. Keep in mind that any single diagnostic test may offer false negative or false positive results, even when it is administered by a professional. If you have a positive reading, you almost certainly will consult a physician, so the problem of such a false reading is not a major one. But a false negative reading may easily lead you to ignore continuing symptoms. Your best course of action, if symptoms persist, is to seek medical help, regardless of a negative test result.

The false negative problem is not a serious one in that category of tests used to monitor a condition. Here, even an occasional error in the test results is not likely to cause difficulty, because the error becomes diluted in the mass of more accurate test readings.

Proponents of do-it-yourself medical testing contend that routine testing done at home to monitor such functions as blood pressure and blood sugar are not only less expensive than are tests done in the physician's office or in hospitals, but may actually be more accurate. If you practice home testing, however, keep in mind that home machines, if they are not carefully calibrated, lose accuracy. In addition, they can be used incorrectly. Check with your doctor about exactly how to use the devices, and the first time you use one, ask your doctor to check out your procedure.

Especially in the case of single-encounter tests, like those for pregnancy, remember that there is always the possibility of false positives and false negatives. A test of this sort should be used mainly as a preliminary screening device. In the case of a positive reading, see a professional to verify your results. In the case of a negative reading, stay alert to symptoms and consult a doctor if there are any indications of a continuing problem.

Above all, remember that the tests don't diagnose. They simply provide some of the information that must be interpreted for a diagnosis to be made. And even those who favor home testing caution about the dangers of self-diagnosis. There's an old saying that anyone who treats himself—a physician included—has a fool for a physician and another for a patient. Even in these days of high-tech computerized machinery on the one hand, and do-it-yourself home testing kits on the other, diagnosis requires more than only a compilation of information.

NEGOTIATING YOUR TESTING PROGRAM

Your own doctor may be a model of the senior partner in the participatory medical decision-making team, sharing with you the information on which he or she bases recommendations and the reasons for decisions, and responding freely to your questions. If so, consider yourself fortunate, indeed, and feel free to ask your questions spontaneously. More likely, however, you'll be dealing with a physician whose ego may be as fragile as yours, and you may very well have a doctor who perceives every question as a challenge. Even as apparently innocent a question as "Do I really need this test?" may evoke an annoyed "If I didn't think you needed it, I wouldn't have ordered it."

Regardless of your doctor's particular personality, if you are to become involved in making medical decisions about your health care, you'll have to ask questions. The key here is to ask them as a participating member of the decision-making team, not as either an adversary or a dependent.

Here are the major categories of testing decisions along with suggested questions.

Those that concern the test itself:

- What can we learn from this test?
- How will the outcome of the test affect my treatment?
- What are the risks involved?
- Is there any other way we can get this information—or any way that is more comfortable, or less costly?

Frequently, doctors fall into the habit of performing certain tests when alternatives exist that may be less risky or less costly. If your doctor recommends an invasive test and you're not satisfied with his answers to your questions about it, get another opinion.

Those that have to do with procedures or timing:

- Are there any special preparations or conditions that I should know about before the test?
- What about eating, drinking liquids, or taking medications?
- What will happen if we wait to do this test?
- Realistically, how long can I wait before we do this test?
- Will the test yield more information if we wait?
- Will the risks increase if we wait?

Be aware that some doctors who have no objection to postponing a test may be concerned about monitoring your condition in the meantime. Even the most cooperative doctor isn't likely to be complacent about the possibility of a malpractice lawsuit for negligence. You might want to make it clear that if you do decide to wait, you intend to exercise your own sense of responsibility by asking:

- If we wait, what should I look for?
- What follow-up measures should I take?
- When should I call your office to report on what's happening, and to whom should I talk?

If you're in a hospital, keep track of the tests that are administered, or ask a family member or other advocate to do so. If it seems to you that you're undergoing an excessive number of tests, or if your blood is being drawn every few hours with no explanation, talk to your doctor.

Those that have to do with test results:

- What do the results mean?
- Should we verify or repeat this test?
- Is there any follow-up procedure in light of the results?
- What should I do now?

If the results are positive, and if a major decision about treatment rides on the accuracy of the test, you should certainly consider a retest—preferably at another lab, and one that is accredited by the College of American Pathologists. Results from such labs tend to be far more accurate than those from uncertified labs. Especially if you believe that the original test was processed in the doctor's— uncertified—office, you can say:

- This is a major decision for me. Shouldn't I have a confirmatory test processed in another laboratory?

Asking the question this way avoids any implication of fault, and provides the doctor with an easy way of agreeing. It's the style we recommend for communicating all of your concerns and questions to your physician, and the one most likely to elicit the information you need.

SUMMING IT ALL UP

Medical testing can be a valuable tool in diagnosis and in monitoring, but test results can be misinterpreted or misused. The more you know about the limitations of testing programs, and of the benefits and risks involved, the more effectively you can participate in making decisions about testing, and the more useful will be the results.

The key principle that should guide you in participating in medical testing decisions is that you should consider the test results in the perspective of your personal concerns, your personal health status, your family history, your age, and your life-style.

As you become more involved in making decisions about medical testing, you should be able to answer each of these questions in the affirmative:

- Do you and your doctor share a common view of the role of medical testing?
- Do you have a fairly clear picture of the benefits and risks that are involved in a particular testing program? If not, can you ask appropriate questions to elicit this information?
- Do you understand the limitations of any tests that your doctor orders for you, the information that will be forthcoming, and the ways in which such information can help in your medical diagnosis or treatment?
- Do you know how to prepare more effectively for the tests to be administered?
- Do you know how to take precautions against the hazards of inappropriate testing, to take account of potential errors in laboratory procedures, and to be aware of possible errors in the interpretation of test results?
- Do you understand the most effective means of following up on test results?

Asking your questions as a participant in the medical decision-making process—rather than as a challenger or a dependent—enhances your doctor's ability to share information and respond candidly to your concerns.

Making Decisions About Treatment

Until recent decades, few choices were available in medical treat-ment. The doctor who diagnosed your condition also treated it, usually with a limited range of medicines and procedures.

The revolutionary advances in medical science have profoundly changed the entire structure of clinical medicine. Medical specialties have proliferated, and diagnostic and treatment options continue to increase. This knowledge explosion in medicine has also fragmented the interests and the views of most physicians. The specialists who are so knowledgeable in their own particular areas of expertise may not be at all well versed in the approaches of alternative specialties.

As a patient who is considering medical treatment, you have two choices. You can put your trust in the doctor's judgment and skill, and your body in his or her hands, hoping for the best, but reserving the right to complain if the outcome is unacceptable. Or you can share in the decision-making process, helping to shape the decisions in what you consider your best interests, but being prepared to accept the risks and responsibilities that accompany autonomy.

BEFORE DECIDING ON TREATMENT

There are few times that the need for treatment is so urgent that options aren't possible. Some emergencies are so obvious that the first order of business is to act fast. When you're rushed to the emergency room, bleeding from an automobile accident, the doctor isn't likely to initiate a discussion of your options, nor are you likely to be interested in anything but life-saving treatment. Among the emergencies that also call for immediate attention are such problems as constant, severe abdominal pain, unrelieved chest pains, or sudden, unexpected deterioration in the state of consciousness.

Fortunately, the vast proportion of medical treatment is not in the category of immediately life-threatening emergencies. Most medical situations allow the time for you and your family to ask questions, consider additional consultation, and weigh choices before you make a major decision. Even some emergency situations may offer time to consider options, after the life-threatening condition has been stabilized. For example, once a heart attack has been dealt with and you're in stable condition, you'll have plenty of time to consider whether you should have a cardiac catheterization, angioplasty, or a coronary artery bypass operation. You'll be able to talk with your family, consult experts, and consider your choices.

The first rule in weighing options is to distinguish between major emergencies that call for immediate treatment and conditions for which treatment can be postponed until you have had a chance to consider alternatives. Ask: "What will happen if I wait?" Only if irreparable harm will result should you give up your right to explore your choices.

Doctors may have reasons of their own to act sooner rather than later. The physician may be an aggressive practitioner whose own personal drive to fix a problem impels him or her to intervene immediately. Or he or she may want early intervention in order to minimize the patient's pain or psychological distress. Then again, perhaps the operating room won't be available for another week if the procedure isn't performed tomorrow. The doctor also may be going out of town for a meeting or a vacation in a few days. If you're already in the hospital after an emergency, many doctors will assume it's most convenient to finish the job before you are released.

Patients are often highly susceptible to recommendations for immediate action. People who face a medical problem have a perfectly natural sense of urgency about acting quickly, and in such situations a doctor's recommendation to do so can be very appealing.

Sometimes the most appropriate treatment involves watchful waiting. Yet a physician's need to take action is often spurred by the patient's expectation that something will be done, or *should* be done. Knowing this dynamic, you might suggest to the doctor that you're willing to postpone any treatment beyond supportive care and observation, if such a course of action is appropriate. This kind of comment may relieve the doctor of the pressure to act on a falsely perceived sense of urgency and free you to explore all your options without unnecessary stress.

WEIGHING TREATMENT OPTIONS

Once you begin to explore choices, you may find that you can choose from among a relatively large array of possibilities, each with its risks, costs, and benefits. On the other hand, you may find that your particular medical problem doesn't offer many, or even any, effective choices. In some cases, there may be no available treatment other than providing as much support and comfort as possible.

Depending on your particular diagnosis, your choice may be fairly easy. One good established approach may exist that's not only effective, but offers minimal risk and expense. There is essentially no controversy about the choice of surgery when someone has an acute appendicitis that threatens to rupture, for example. However, in most cases, you're more likely to have to weigh the alternatives in terms of the effectiveness of the treatment (which you'll find out about by asking questions of your doctor or doctors) and your own evaluation of the risks and costs.

The great majority of medical problems do offer choices. Many problems may be treated either with surgery or with drugs, for example. Even if surgery is the only feasible choice, there are often several procedures that might be considered. The same is usually true when medication is the recommended form of treatment.

Are the Results Reversible?

In narrowing down your choices, consider that some treatments are reversible and some are not. Many drugs, for example, have no significant lasting effect, and you can try them to see if they work for you. While risks are involved in virtually every form of treatment, whether or not they materialize usually becomes apparent over time, with a parallel opportunity to stop or correct the treatment. On the other hand, once an organ has been removed, it can't be replaced, and some procedures result in scars or mutilation, unpleasant physical consequences, or psychological trauma. When you discuss options with your doctor, consider whether the effects of the treatment are reversible or whether there is no turning back once you have reached a particular stage of therapy.

What Are the Risks, Costs, and Benefits for *You*?

Begin with the understanding that the only "good" choice in medicine is to stay healthy. Once you have a problem, all of your choices will involve trade-offs between your costs and risks on the one hand, and the projected benefits on the other. Some of the costs are virtual certainties, while many risks and benefits are possibilities that can be evaluated only in terms of odds. The costs may include money, risks of death or injury, pain and suffering, stress, or a combination of any of these. The benefits can range from the temporary relief or cure of a problem to the prevention of an even worse problem. Your choices may not range between good and bad; often you will be presented with choosing between bad and worse. In making your decision, you should choose what *you* perceive as the least of the possible evils, taking into account the costs and the benefits of the alternatives.

One of the problems is that if your condition is serious, your primary-care physician may not want to be the bearer of bad news, and he or she may not volunteer all of the negative possibilities. You'll be apprised of the problem, of course, for withholding this kind of information constitutes malpractice. You'll also probably be offered a number of options. But the physician may be reluctant to let you know his or her own estimate of the relative disadvantages of each—unless you ask directly. If you have confidence in your doctor, you should ask, "What choice would *you* make if you were in my position. Why?" Consider the doctor's response along with the rest of the information you'll gather before you make your decision.

When you consult a specialist, you'll face a very different problem. Keep in mind that surgeons or radiation therapists explain risks and benefits in terms of their own perspective about the choices and not necessarily in terms of yours, and that every specialist is biased. Moreover, remember that most doctors are more comfortable discussing quantifiable data about taking risks and are less comfortable discussing such ambiguities as "quality of life." Doctors are likely to have definite opinions on whether the risks are justified, and they tend to be enthusiastic about the benefits of the services they offer because they believe in what they do. But it's you who will bear the costs and you who will live with the results. You have the ultimate responsibility for deciding if the risks and costs outweigh the benefits for any suggested treatment.

It may be difficult to cast the calculations in terms of what is best for you, and the ways the risks are presented may heavily influence your own perception. For example, if the doctor tells you that a particular procedure has an 80 percent chance of success, you're likely to perceive the odds very differently than if you're told that there is a 20 percent chance of failure. (See chapter 3.)

Take your time in gathering information, in ordering your own priorities, and in evaluating both the risks and costs, and the benefits. The ultimate question will be: Are the possible benefits worth the costs and the risks? To repeat: Don't be rushed into a decision. But do set a reasonable time limit within which to decide, even if what you decide is to forgo treatment; it's unrealistic to decide to put off a treatment decision until a miracle cure comes along.

Which Specialty?

Self-diagnosis and self-referral to a specialist can themselves be risky. Unless you've had previous contact with a specialist and know just what your problem is, you face the hazard of choosing an inappropriate specialty. We noted earlier that patients who seek out a specialist put themselves in the hands of doctors who are predisposed to find the problems they expect to find and to treat these problems according to their training. In the narrowed world of specialty, a cardiologist may see a heart problem where an allergist may see an allergic reaction. Calling the local medical society or a hospital with a sound reputation may provide the names of qualified specialists, but it won't help you if your self-diagnosis has fallen short.

Information-gathering should usually begin with your primary-care physician, who has your medical records and who is most likely to know your medical history. He or she will certainly make a tentative diagnosis and will probably do some preliminary testing. Perhaps he or she already has tried some conservative (nonsurgical, for example) treatments before steering you to a specialist for further testing or for treatment. You're under no obligation to accept the specific recommendation of your primary-care doctor, but if you have confidence in him or her, the recommendation is probably better than any you would get from a friend or neighbor, or even from the local medical society.

WATCHFUL WAITING

We commented earlier that Americans have a propensity to view the body as a machine that needs to be "fixed" when a problem develops; patients want the doctor to "do something." One highly respectable and successful form of medical treatment is often misinterpreted as doing nothing: a course of supportive care and careful observation. What this means is that the doctor and the patient agree to postpone intervention with active treatment until it is clear that treatment is called for, while the doctor acts to relieve any discomfort that may occur and takes measures to prevent further damage.

There is always the possibility that intervention may do more harm than good, thus violating medicine's major tenet of *Primum non nocere*. In a variety of situations, it's possible that no intervention—medicines, surgery, radiation therapy, or any other treatment—is likely to improve the body's ability to heal itself. Sometimes patients assume the costs and risks of intervention in such cases without reasonable expectation of benefit.

A simple example: Patients often ask doctors for antibiotics to treat the common cold. Yet, with or without antibiotics, a cold will normally last about a week, and those patients who take antibiotics expose themselves to unnecessary costs and risks, with no real benefit. Sometimes the cause of the infection may not be clear; bacterial infections can be helped by antibiotics, while viral infections can't be. Most often, the nature of the infection becomes clear with time, however, and the patient who is willing to live with a degree of uncertainty may avoid the greater costs and risks of unnecessary medication.

Another common example is furnished by the case of a woman with fibroids—benign muscular tumors in the wall of the uterus—who is approaching menopause. Fibroids may periodically cause heavy bleeding, and the problem can be resolved quickly with a hysterectomy—the surgical removal of the uterus. A possible alternative is to try controlling the bleeding with medication until menopause is reached, at which time the fibroids are more likely to shrink by themselves.

You must decide for yourself how you feel about taking risks and how well you can handle ambiguity and uncertainty. Is it more important to have an early resolution of the problem, even at the expense of the risks and costs involved? Or is it more important for you to avoid or postpone the risks, considering the possibility that the problem may resolve itself or that the decision will become clearer with time?

Keeping in mind your own feelings about risks and uncertainty, you might want to ask the doctor:

- What can I lose and what can I gain by waiting? Will there be irreparable harm if I wait?
- Is the problem likely to go away by itself? If so, under what conditions and in what period of time?
- Will the nature of the problem become clearer if I wait?
- Can the discomfort or the symptoms be controlled if I decide not to go ahead with the treatment you propose?
- What are the risks and the likelihood of benefit with the procedure?

Again, keep in mind that specialists set great store in the therapeutic value of their specialties. If you feel that you're being pressured into an operation about which you have serious reservations, get another opinion.

PRESCRIPTION MEDICINES

The traditional medical visit often concludes with a ritual in which the doctor hands the patient a piece of paper with the symbol of the potion that will relieve pain, restore vitality, or cure disease. Many patients think that unless the doctor writes a prescription, no "treatment" of the problem has been addressed. A 1988 report by the subcommittee on clinical pharmacology of the American College of Physicians, noting that approximately two-thirds of all medical visits involve a prescription, concluded that a good deal of drug therapy is overdone. Among the subcommittee's findings: Three in five physicians prescribed antibiotics for the common cold, and in hospitals up to two-thirds of prescribed antibiotics may have been unnecessary or inappropriately administered.

The subcommittee described a "drug revolution" in the United States and noted that a new chemical was being approved for human use on the average of once every three weeks. And the increase in the use of prescription drugs was bringing a corresponding increase in adverse reactions, many of which, according to the subcommittee, could have been prevented by more prudent use of medications.

While you may not think of it in those terms, you make a treatment decision every time you take a pill or a tablet, even if it's something as apparently innocuous as aspirin or vitamins.

Will the Drug Do More Good Than Harm?

You and your doctor will have to balance a number of separate factors in deciding whether or not you should use a particular drug. Be aware that your doctor's ranking of the importance of the following elements in terms of costs and benefits may or may not match yours. The factors are:

Efficacy. Does the drug do what it's supposed to do, and will it do any good for you? Both you and your doctor are likely to consider this a major factor in choosing a drug. To the doctor, it will probably be the primary factor.

Side effects and risks. Remember that there is no absolutely safe drug. You and your doctor are likely to agree that unwanted side effects may be a problem, but your own view of such side effects may differ from the doctor's. You'll both be concerned about those that may be *permanent* and that are referred to as risks, like deafness, kidney failure, and even death. But you are likely to be far more concerned than the doctor about side effects that probably will disappear when you stop taking the drug, such as dizziness, rashes, nausea, stomach aches, or drowsiness. If you experience side effects from a medication, ask the doctor whether they represent a *threat* to your health or whether they should be considered merely *annoyances*.

Because drugs don't affect everyone in precisely the same way, you may experience unexpected side effects even if you take the drug as it has been prescribed. You'll have to be the judge of how much discomfort you're willing to tolerate in terms of temporary side effects that can be classified as annoying. Regardless of your tolerance, however, don't suffer silently if a drug bothers you. The doctor may reduce the dosage or may be able to substitute another drug, because both the benefits and the side effects may vary widely from drug to drug, even in the same group of medications.

Some medications may not produce therapeutic effects until after they have been taken for several weeks, even though side effects may be apparent early. For example, tricyclic antidepressants such as desipramine will cause dry mouth within 24 hours after you have begun taking them, but a therapeutic response may not be seen for weeks, even when the dose is appropriate. Often simply knowing what to expect in the way of unpleasant effects can enable you to tolerate a potentially useful medication without abandoning it prematurely.

Health-threatening side effects from medications may show up in blood tests long before symptoms of severe or permanent damage are apparent. The sometimes irreversible kidney damage caused in some cases by two aminoglycoside antibiotics, gentamicin and tobramycin, is detectable and preventable by monitoring with appropriate blood tests, for example. When you ask the doctor about risks or adverse effects of medications, ask whether you will need any laboratory tests or other monitoring to detect problems early, before serious damage is done.

Cost and quality. The doctor is likely to be concerned with quality far more than with cost. In fact, many doctors don't even know the cost of prescription drugs in their own communities. In the absence of specific information, the doctor may prescribe a brand-name drug rather than a less expensive generic drug. While the brand-name drug and the generic are chemical equivalents, they may not have precisely the same effects. The Food and Drug Administration, which approves prescription drugs, contends that such differences are negligible, but most doctors distrust automatic substitutions because of variations in patients' response. If your doctor prescribes a brand name, you might ask both the doctor and your pharmacist if a less expensive generic will do as well.

Administering the drug. You certainly should consider such issues as the frequency with which you'll have to take the drug, how convenient it is to take, and how long you'll have to take it. These are also issues that are likely to concern you far more than they'll concern the doctor. In some cases, the most effective drugs are those most inconvenient or difficult to take. For example, a diabetic who can't control his or her blood sugar with oral agents (pills) may have to consider insulin. The problem is that insulin can be taken only by injection, so the patient may have to decide whether the inconvenience is acceptable in order to achieve greater control over blood sugar and the long-term effects that high blood sugar can cause: kidney damage, nerve damage, and accelerated atherosclerosis. Once such long-term damage is apparent, it's usually too late to reverse or correct it. To the doctor, the choice is clear: control the blood sugar to help avoid the damage from diabetes. But to some patients, the side effects and inconvenience of insulin therapy may be too high a price to pay for the possibility of benefits years in the future. Even if the choices don't involve questions of efficacy, there may still be trade-offs of convenience or personal preference about the form of drug—pill or liquid, for example.

Questions you should ask:

- How effective is the drug?
- What risks or side effects are possible?
- Do I have choices in the way the drug is administered?
- Is there a reason I shouldn't use a generic alternative?
- Do I take the drug on an empty stomach or with food?
- Do I have to take the medication at any special time?
- How long will I need to take the medication?
- Does it interact with any of my other medication?

Drug Combinations and Interactions

Decisions become far more complex when you are taking medication for more than one problem. Different drugs can interact in a variety of ways. One can increase the effects (either therapeutic or adverse) of the other or can minimize or even neutralize them.

For example, the aspirin that someone takes for arthritis will increase the activity of the blood-thinning drug warfarin (Coumadin). The anti-ulcer medication cimetidine (Tagamet) can inhibit the liver's removal of such drugs as theophylline, used to ease respiratory problems, and the tranquilizer diazepam (Valium), thereby increasing their effects. On the other hand, barbiturates and nicotine enhance the liver's ability to metabolize the same drugs, thus necessitating larger doses to achieve desired therapeutic effects. The direct stomach irritation caused by the antibiotic erythromycin together with the anti-inflammatory agent ibuprofen (Advil, Nuprin) can result in heartburn or pain that neither alone would cause. And some substances may simply interfere with the absorption of drugs from the stomach. That's the reason why antacids should not be given at the same time as the antibiotic tetracycline.

When the doctor prescribes a drug, tell (or remind) him or her about other drugs you're taking and ask about potential interactions. Not only prescribed drugs, but alcohol that you drink and tobacco that you smoke may interact with medications in harmful ways, so be sure to ask either your doctor or your pharmacist about possible interactions.

Monitoring Your Treatment

Obviously, you expect that your medication treatment will help you get better and won't make you worse. Since you're the one who will be taking the medicine, you're often in the best position to report on the results.

However, sometimes the effects—both bad and good—won't be readily apparent. If you take medication for high blood pressure, you'll know if it's working only by measuring your blood pressure with a sphygmomanometer. For example, you won't know if the diuretic you're taking to reduce blood pressure by lowering the amount of water in the body is also causing too much potassium loss or if the angiotensin converting enzyme (ACE) inhibitors captopril and enalopril are interfering with your kidney function unless you take blood tests. You should ask the doctor about what monitoring you can do and what should be done about those effects you can't detect yourself.

We noted that sometimes expected side effects show up long before a medication has beneficial results. If you know about them in advance, you won't give up a treatment before the drug works as it should.

Some of the questions to ask:

- How long will it take for effects to show up?
- Will I be able to monitor the drug program myself? If not, how can we know if it's working properly?
- Which side effects are "normal" and which are danger signals?

Drug Substitutions

The issue of drug substitutions is based squarely on the relative costs of drugs, and the issue of costs is often either not sufficiently appreciated or simply ignored by physicians. This unfortunate insulation from economic reality is enhanced by the fact that patients may complain to each other, but they rarely express concern to the doctor about the high cost of prescriptions. In medical school, costs are seldom discussed; the emphasis is on the efficacy and the risks of medications. Unless doctors or members of their family are sick, physicians may have little awareness of the cost of medications. And even then, the doctors will usually obtain medications at a discount, or even free from a pharmaceutical company representative.

The substitution of other kinds of drugs (therapeutic substitution) or of lower-priced equivalents for brand-name products (generic substitution) may be highly justified if the substitute is as effective (or even almost as effective) as the original prescription.

Therapeutic substitution means that one *kind* of drug has been substituted for another because it provides the same, or nearly the same, benefit at a significantly lower cost. This kind of substitution is rarely brought to the attention of the public, because until recently it usually has been practiced only in hospitals, which can save considerably by such a change. There the decision about therapeutic equivalence is made by special committees composed of doctors and pharmacists, in accordance with standards established by the Joint Committee on Hospital Accreditation.

Therapeutic substitution is also practiced at some outpatient pharmacies that are associated with HMOs. One study found that 30 percent of the 187 responding HMOs had pharmacy plans that permitted therapeutic substitutions, and one central Michigan HMO was able to save $1 million in 1987 through such substitutions. Yet outside of HMOs and the outpatient services of the Veterans Administration hospitals, the practice isn't widespread.

Such substitution is controversial when it is practiced on an outpatient basis without the controls that are mandated for hospitals. Some types of medications can present idiosyncratic variations. For example, the arthritis drugs ibuprofen (Motrin) and naproxen (Naprosyn) differ in cost, efficacy, dosing frequency, and—for some people—the intensity of gastrointestinal side effects. However, since they are both nonsteroidal anti-inflammatory drugs (of which more than a dozen are on the market), they are interchanged in some situations. If you are in a treatment situation that permits or mandates therapeutic substitution, ask the doctor if such substitution will make any significant difference in your case. More important, if the medication you take doesn't seem to be working, or if you experience side effects, ask the doctor if either condition might be the result of therapeutic substitution. The doctor may not even be aware of such a substitution, so bring the drug container to the office so that he or she can examine it.

Generic substitution means that a chemically equivalent drug is substituted for a brand-name product. Some inexpensive drugs may work as well as the original and some may not. There may be differences in the rates at which the substances are absorbed into the system, for example. It's because of these differences that some states don't permit pharmacists automatically to substitute generics for certain categories of brand-name products, unless the doctor prescribes the generic specifically.

The doctor may not always be aware when a brand-name prescription has been filled with a generic drug. If you are not responding to a medication, especially if that medication was effective in the past, bring the pills or the container to the doctor and ask whether the use of the brand-name drug would be more effective. However, many generic drugs work as well as the original brand-name product. If you are concerned about costs, ask your doctor if a less expensive equivalent would be satisfactory (see chapter 5).

MAKING DECISIONS ABOUT SURGERY

The decision about whether to have surgery probably causes more anxiety than does any other medical decision. Not only are surgical procedures among the most risky in the medical cornucopia, but they usually cause more discomfort than medical (nonsurgical) treatments, and they are almost always more expensive.

One of the more anxiety-causing elements is the knowledge that the results of surgery are rarely reversible. When an organ or tissue is removed, it's gone forever. Even when replacement parts such as artificial joints, blood vessels, and heart valves wear out, they are difficult to replace, because the initial implantation causes scarring and adhesions that make repeated procedures much more difficult to perform successfully. For all practical purposes, once an operation is performed, the process can't be reversed.

Is the Surgery Needed?

You need to address three important questions when you consider surgery:

- What is the surgery intended to accomplish?
- What is likely to happen if you don't have it?
- What alternatives do you have?

The answers are likely to differ substantially if you are considering a type of surgery that could save your life or remove an immediate threat to your health, rather than discretionary surgery aimed at improving the quality of your life.

Emergency surgery, or surgery that deals with an immediate threat, may be unavoidable, because if it isn't performed, the consequences can be far more serious than the effects and risks of the surgery itself. When the blood flow is so reduced that you're in danger of losing an organ or a limb, there may be no good alternative to cleaning out the artery or implanting a new blood vessel to provide circulation. When cancer threatens a major organ, surgery may be the only reasonable approach to save the organ and possibly your life.

However, a good deal of surgery is discretionary, or "elective." This includes the surgical procedures that may be performed to reduce symptoms or to improve a particular body function. Cataract surgery will do both; so will hip-replacement surgery. The decision is based on a value choice: Is the expected improvement worth the risks and costs of the surgery?

In a different category is preventive surgery, the purpose of which is to prevent future risk, disability, or death. The need for preventive surgery is based on the weighing of probabilities. If nothing is done, does the likelihood of damage outweigh the costs and risks of surgery?

Such procedures as coronary artery bypass surgery and coronary angioplasty are used in part to reduce angina pains, but also to lower the risks of future heart attacks. Both procedures focus on those areas of the coronary arteries that have been identified by angiography as sites of present and probable later obstruction. A 1988 study by Dr. William C. Little and his colleagues at the Bowman Gray School of Medicine of Wake Forest University raised questions about the rationale for some of these preventive procedures. They found that when they examined coronary angiograms done on people who *later* had heart attacks, the most severe blockages visible on the X rays were not necessarily the ones that caused the later heart damage. The doctors simply could not have predicted specifically where or when the heart-muscle damage would have occurred by using the angiogram.

Clinical investigators, economists, and statisticians have attempted to assess the relative value of other forms of preventive surgery. Rarely have their findings been clear and unequivocal.

Carotid endarterectomy, for example, is an operation that is performed to prevent strokes that might result from a total blockage of blood flow or from a cholesterol plaque dislodged from the inside of one of the carotid arteries in the neck. An estimated 107,000 carotid endarterectomies were performed in this country in 1985, according to the National Center for Health Statistics. The figure was seven times the number performed in 1971. Researchers at the Rand Corporation convened panels of distinguished physicians in 1986 to identify criteria and standards for determining when such surgery is appropriate.

When Dr. Constance Winslow and her colleagues at the Rand Corporation applied these criteria to a group of 1,302 patients in three geographic areas, they concluded that about one-third of the patients had been given a carotid endarterectomy for appropriate reasons, one-third for questionable reasons, and one-third for inappropriate reasons. Their conclusion was that in many cases this form of surgery was "substantially overused."

Moreover, the expert physicians who had developed the standards agreed on only half of the specific criteria. More to the point, they disagreed on about 20 percent of the standards—and that was *after* they had discussed the criteria together.

While such studies make it clear that surgical procedures may be performed inappropriately, they also show that experts can disagree on the specific criteria for making a surgical decision. And, as we noted earlier, the differences in the rates at which some operations are performed may vary dramatically from one locality to another, apparently reflecting local practice rather than any scientifically justifiable rationale.

One interesting note: In the Rand Corporation study, even after the discussions of the various criteria for surgery had taken place, a greater number of surgeons than nonsurgeons (including medical specialists and generalists) on the panel consistently felt that surgery was more appropriate.

This points up the importance of exploring the need for surgery first with your primary-care physician. Your own doctor, assuming that he or she is not a surgeon, is far less likely to be as biased toward or as enthusiastic about surgery as is a surgeon, and is far more likely to have considered the possibility of treatment with medication. If your own doctor suggests surgery, ask:

- Why are you recommending surgery?
- What specific procedure are you suggesting?
- What is likely to happen if I don't have surgery?
- If I wait, could I decide to have the operation at a later date?
- Are there any reasonable alternatives to this surgery?

The primary-care doctor may not be able to answer all these questions and may suggest that you ask the surgeon (or another specialist, if you explore alternatives). If that is the case, your own doctor may be able to help you develop a set of appropriate questions to ask.

Sometimes the recommendation for surgery will come from a surgeon, such as a gynecologist, who is also in a primary-care role, and this can place the patient in an awkward situation. If you want an additional diagnostic opinion, or if you want to consider other surgeons, just tell the doctor that you want to be absolutely sure before you make such an important decision. A patient's primary allegiance should be to himself or herself, and this self-interest overrides any concern about the doctor's feelings or ego.

Choosing a Surgeon

Once you decide on surgery, you have to pick a surgeon. This can be a stressful process, because a surgeon's mistakes may be difficult or impossible to rectify.

Let's start with ways in which you should *not* choose a surgeon. One is to rely solely on recommendations from friends and relatives. Unfortunately, having survived an operation with no complications doesn't make someone an authority on judging the competence of a surgeon. However, friends and relatives can tell you a good deal about how well the surgeon communicated with them and how competently he or she handled the postoperative care.

Certainly, you shouldn't rely on the yellow pages for corroboration of specialty training. A survey in Hartford, Connecticut, showed that one out of eight physicians listed in that city's phone directory under a specialist category wasn't board-certified.

The most appropriate person to ask first is your primary-care doctor. If the operation is a common or routine one, your search for a surgeon may not need to extend beyond your immediate geographic area. Since he or she is likely to be familiar with the local medical community, your primary-care physician should be able to recommend several competent surgeons. In a large metropolitan area, this local medical community may consist of a single hospital or, in a nonurban setting, an entire region.

Ask your doctor to suggest the names of several surgeons in the appropriate field whom the doctor would trust to operate on him or her or on a family member. Ask carefully about each surgeon's experience. How many operations like yours does the surgeon perform each year?

Experience is important. A study from the New York State Department of Health that was published in the *Journal of the American Medical Association* in 1989 confirmed that there is an inverse relationship between the number of times a surgeon performs a specific operation or the number of such operations at a particular hospital, and the mortality rates for that surgeon and that hospital. Your own doctor may or may not know the actual extent of the surgeon's experience, complication rate, or mortality rate, but ask anyway. Also ask the doctor how well he or she knows the surgeon, because if the relationship is a close social one, as opposed to a solely professional one, you may want more objective information before you make your decision.

Once the doctor gives you several names of surgeons, ask what factors differentiate them. Is it a matter of personality, or is it more a matter of proficiency and approach? Is one more aggressive and another more deliberate in his or her willingness to perform surgery? Patterns of practice may vary from city to city, and even from hospital to hospital in the same locale. More important, however, is the difference in practice patterns between physicians in the same hospital. For example, obstetrician Dr. Gregory Goyert and his colleagues from the Wayne State University Medical School found that the rate of cesarean section deliveries varied between 19 percent and 42 percent among obstetricians in a single community hospital. After examining the variables involved, Dr. Goyert concluded that the variation was attributable only to the preferences and practice patterns of the individual physicians.

For a particularly serious or unusual problem, you may wish to broaden your search for a surgeon. That doesn't mean that you may not find excellent care close to home, but don't hesitate to look elsewhere in order to be as certain as you can that you will be getting the care you need. Going to a large medical center is not necessarily a guarantee of engaging the most able surgeon. In fact, for relatively common operations such as cholecystectomy or total hip replacement, or for major procedures that are commonly performed, such as coronary artery bypass procedures in patients without complicated problems, the experience at a large community hospital can easily equal that of major medical centers. However, for procedures that are performed infrequently or that are on the cutting edge of technology, you're likely to find the surgeons with the greatest experience in university medical centers. If you know physicians elsewhere, or if family members or friends have contacts in other medical communities, ask them about resources in their communities. Most important, be as persistent in your search as you feel you need to be, because no one else is likely to be as forceful an advocate as you will be for yourself. Finding the right surgeon can be a hit-or-miss procedure, and if you're not satisfied with the advice and choices that you've been given, it may be best to wait, as long as waiting won't immediately affect your overall health.

Finally, check out the hospital. Surgeons may be the stars, but the quality of the operation will depend to a great extent on the quality of the surgical team—the anesthesiologist, the nurses, and the technicians. Like surgeons, hospitals have track records that depend in large part on their experience in performing the kinds of operation that you'll undergo. There are remarkable differences in hospital death rates for the same operation, and the track records for hospitals are readily available.

First, hospitals keep records, and the administrators know how well or poorly they perform particular operations. In fact, many hospitals now brag in their advertisements if they have low mortality rates. Even if you can't get the information from the hospital, ask your primary-care doctor. If that's not productive, you may obtain the Medicare mortality data for that hospital from the Health Care Financing Administration in Washington, D.C., by calling (202) 727-0735, or by contacting the nearest regional office of the Department of Health and Human Services. Although mortality data can vary according to how sick the patients at a hospital are, it does allow a rough comparison of facilities.

While many insurance companies encourage and even mandate additional opinions on the need for surgery, if you are enrolled in an HMO there may be restrictions on whom you can consult. HMOs may offer only a limited number of such surgical specialists as orthopedists and neurosurgeons, and if you are not satisfied with the choices available, you may be forced to assume part or all of the bill for an additional opinion or for the operation itself. When you are sick and admitted to the hospital, your illness and your confinement may also narrow your range of choices, especially if you are so ill that surgery can't be delayed. In this case, you can only hope that your family or friends will be your vigorous advocates and that your doctor will act with your best interests in mind.

Talking with the Surgeon

Before you meet the surgeon, do your homework. Find out where the surgeon trained and whether he or she is board-certified. The referring doctor may know or can look up the information for you. You can also check with the medical staff office or the department of surgery at the hospital. Check the *Directory of Medical Specialists*, which may be available at your public library, and certainly will be in the library of the closest public hospital. This reference book will give you the relevant biographical information.

When you see the surgeon, unless you are absolutely convinced of the need for the operation, the first matter you should ask about is the necessity for surgery. Does the surgeon agree with the recommendation for surgery, and if so, why? If not, why not? Ask him or her to list the specific reasons, and write them down. In addition, ask for the surgeon's prediction of what would happen if you choose not to have the operation; as we noted, you always have the option of waiting, unless irreparable harm will be done.

You should also ask the surgeon for detailed information about the proposed procedure itself. Where will it be performed? Many procedures are now performed in outpatient surgical units and doctors' offices, although surgery that requires any significant postoperative care or monitoring will probably be performed inside a hospital. Will the operation require a general anesthetic, and if so, will there be a choice? A spinal anesthetic (your lower body is totally numbed but you remain awake) facilitates a faster recovery. Unfortunately, for operations that involve any part of the body above the pelvic cavity, spinal anesthesia is not an available option.

Most candidates for surgery overlook the importance of anesthesia, considering it merely a procedural detail. But for many surgical procedures, the anesthesia presents the major risk for the operation. You should ask the surgeon to let you know who will be administering the anesthesia and what his or her qualifications are. Find out whether the surgeon prefers to work with one anesthesiologist rather than another. If, on the basis of previous experiences or reports from others, you have strong negative feelings about the anesthesiologist, offer to alter your schedule to accommodate the availability of another anesthesiologist.

Ask the surgeon to describe the actual procedure to be performed in a sequence of steps, and ask him or her to make drawings so that you can review them later. Having a clear understanding of the proposed operation allows you to feel at least some degree of control at a time when your feelings of vulnerability will be strong. Ask the doctor how you're likely to feel after the surgery, on a day-by-day basis, for three or four days after the operation. Simply knowing what to expect removes some of the aura of mystery that surrounds surgical procedures and will enable you to cope more fully.

Once you have a clear idea about the need for surgery and you understand what the process entails, ask the doctor about the likelihood for success. Is success measured in all-or-none terms or is there a spectrum of outcomes ranging between good and bad? Surgery to treat cancer, for example, may not be considered successful unless all of the cancerous tissue is removed, while surgery to restore movement to the hip may result in varying degrees of success that range from a full or partial restoration of function to no benefit at all.

Since some procedures don't produce immediate benefits, ask if you can expect a lag or delay in seeing the full benefits of the surgery. The effects of cosmetic surgery will probably be masked initially by swelling or bleeding in the involved tissues. Joint replacements are also complicated by swelling due to the surgical process, and the extent of postsurgical joint function may not be fully apparent for weeks.

Ask about risks. What complications may occur during the surgery? What are the long-term risks, the chances that you'll end up with a problem—a disability or disease—that you didn't have before? And ask about the statistics involved: What are the odds that you will suffer damage? How is success measured, and what is the rate of success for this particular procedure? What is the doctor's own record of success—and the hospital's? The surgeon should be able to provide you with objective statistics on complications and death. Ask specifically if the doctor has data on how well his or her own surgical patients fared after leaving the hospital. When Dr. John E. Wennberg of Dartmouth College Medical School and his colleagues established the Maine Medical Assessment Project (see chapter 1), they found that few doctors tried to follow up on their own patients. And even though you've already asked your primary-care doctor, ask the surgeon what you can expect if you choose not to have the surgery. Then you can weigh the risks of the surgery against the risks of watchful waiting.

Ask about the expected aftercare. What will be the extent of your disability after the surgery, and will there be any way for you to speed up the process of recuperation? Exercises can prevent the loss of muscle tone and sometimes reduce the risks of postoperative blood clots. If there's a special activity that you like to engage in regularly, ask the surgeon how long you're likely to wait after the operation before being able to resume it.

Variations in Cost

The costs of specific surgical procedures can vary tremendously from one surgeon to another, and you don't always get what you pay for. A survey commissioned by Ryder Trucks in Miami found that the area's board-certified physicians actually charged considerably lower fees than those who were not board-certified. Before you make your final arrangements, ask the surgeon whether he or she will accept your insurance reimbursement as payment in full or whether there will be an additional charge. If you settle these issues before surgery, you can avoid later misunderstandings and ill will.

Invasive Therapeutic Procedures

With the development of newer ways to gain access into the body, the boundaries between traditional surgical specialists and medical specialists who use invasive techniques have become increasingly blurred. A new hybrid specialist is developing, one who performs the diagnostic testing to determine the need for treatment and then the therapeutic procedure itself. Occasionally, both are combined in a single procedure, using the same equipment. The invasive therapeutic procedures offer many advantages over traditional surgery, but caution is still in order.

Colonoscopy, for example, involves the use of an approximately five-foot-long fiber optic scope that is inserted through the anal opening to examine the colon. If polyps are found, they can be removed and subsequently examined for malignancy without additional surgery. Coronary angioplasty is performed by inserting a catheter through a small puncture wound, usually in the groin. Using this method, the cardiologist may be able to clear blocked arteries by expanding a "balloon" in the artery. Arthroscopic and laparoscopic procedures involve the insertion of special instruments through tiny incisions in the joint or abdomen to remove or repair damaged tissue or, in the case of laparoscopy, to perform tubal ligations for sterilization.

Such invasive medical procedures have certain major advantages over traditional surgery. People who undergo them usually require either little sedation or only brief general anesthesia. These particular procedures replace surgical operations that are much more expensive and painful and that can cause persistent scarring, both internally and externally. The patient is able to walk out of the hospital or surgical facility either the same day or, in the case of coronary angioplasty, after 24 to 48 hours of observation. One of the most dramatic demonstrations of the success of such procedures is the case of Joan Benoit, who underwent arthroscopic knee surgery and then won the Olympic Trials Marathon race just six weeks afterward.

Despite such benefits, these procedures aren't without risks and drawbacks. Colonoscopy can result in a perforated colon. Coronary angioplasty may cause spasms of the artery, necessitating urgent coronary bypass surgery. Such complications are infrequent, but they may require an immediate operation to control the damage. In addition, certain circumstances may limit their use. Some of the techniques require working with small instruments within areas of the body that are relatively confined. As a result, these techniques are useful only if they are performed within a limited, well-defined range. If there is more extensive involvement, surgery may be necessary. For example, if there are multiple blocked areas in a blood vessel or if the multiple vessels are obstructed, the invasive angioplasty may have to be repeated several times, or other surgical intervention may be required. The physical and financial costs of repeated invasive procedures can add up to greater temporary disability and expense than would result from one larger surgical operation.

Nevertheless, technological advances occur rapidly—a fact that leads to still another potential problem. While the range of what can be accomplished with invasive procedures is rapidly expanding, there is always pressure from the public on the specialists and their colleagues to use newer invasive techniques before they are fully validated.

That these procedures are both diagnostic and then therapeutic makes for efficient treatment. But it can also greatly reduce patient participation in making decisions. Once the procedure is under way, the specialist makes the determination to perform a further procedure based on what he or she sees during the investigation. Because the same person diagnoses, makes a decision about need, and then performs the procedure, an important check and balance in the therapeutic process is lost. Moreover, the patient is given little or no time to consider choices when the doctor says, "There's a blockage here that I can fix. Should I go ahead and do it?"

Because this sequence virtually eliminates the patient from on-the-spot deliberating, you should have an absolutely clear understanding of what can be accomplished by an invasive therapeutic procedure before you get started. First, ask the specialist about the "contingency plans" for dealing with whatever problems might be found. Make sure you understand the benefits and risks of any such procedure and how well it meets your medical needs. If you want to be cautious and undergo the procedure only for diagnosis, be clear about the fact that you may need to repeat it if therapy is required, and make certain that the specialist knows your wishes. This one-stage procedure may be appropriate, but remember that you may need a second general anesthesia or arterial puncture if you undertake the second step in the future.

In considering such procedures, you should choose the cardiologist, gastroenterologist, orthopedist, or obstetrician-gynecologist with the same care that you would use to choose a surgeon for an operation. Find out beforehand or at the beginning of a consultation whether the specialist performs invasive therapeutic procedures, and if so, for which problems. Ask about his or her track record for success and complications, as well as all of the questions that you would use to make a decision about your surgeon. Most important, unless you face the immediate threat of death or disability, don't let yourself be rushed into a decision. The time to consider your options and contingencies is *before* you start, not once the procedure is in progress.

COMMON INVASIVE THERAPEUTIC PROCEDURES AND ALTERNATIVES

Procedure	Indications for Therapy	Expected Benefits	Risks	Special Considerations	When to Consider Alternatives	Alternatives
TWELVE SURGICAL PROCEDURES						
Carotid endarterectomy ("cleaning out" the arteries in the front of the neck)	Transient stroke symptoms or visual loss and the presence of significant atherosclerotic plaque in the carotid artery supplying the affected side of the brain. Possible indication: 90% or greater blockage in either carotid artery or lesser blockage with rough-appearing plaque, but without symptoms.	Prevention of transient stroke symptoms, as well as the prevention of future stroke. Prevention of stroke or visual loss caused by a blood clot to the eye.	Small risk from general anesthesia. Modest risk of stroke from the procedure.	The risk of a stroke without surgery is 4%. If the surgeon's rate of complicating stroke exceeds 4%, surgery is not justified.	If the risks of general anesthesia are excessive, or if you feel the risk of stroke does not justify the surgery.	Risk factor reduction: stop smoking, control blood pressure, lower cholesterol. Medication: aspirin and dipyridamole (Persantine).
Cholecystectomy (removal of the gall bladder)	Acute cholecystitis (inflamed gall bladder) that is progressing, threatening rupture, or failing to resolve. Gallstones with accompanying symptoms: recurring pain, transient blockage of bile ducts (sometimes causing inflamed pancreas). Possible indication: presence of multiple small stones.	Cure the acute inflammation and prevent rupture. Prevent bile duct blockage and prevent future cholecystitis. Prevent bile duct blockage and prevent future cholecystitis.	Small risk from general anesthesia and from surgery itself.	Risk of surgery greater in the setting of an acute attack. There may be difficulty digesting fatty foods after the gall bladder is removed.	If the risks of general anesthesia and abdominal surgery are excessive, because of complicating medical conditions or illness.	Medication: may dissolve gall stones, but they reform when Rx is stopped. Risk factor reduction: lower the cholesterol level. Other: shock wave breakup of stones is experimental.

COMMON INVASIVE THERAPEUTIC PROCEDURES AND ALTERNATIVES *(continued)*

Procedure	Indications for Therapy	Expected Benefits	Risks	Special Considerations	When to Consider Alternatives	Alternatives
Coronary artery bypass (inserting new blood vessels to improve blood flow to the heart muscle)	Chronic stable angina with symptoms despite taking medication, or inability to tolerate medication.	Relief of angina in more than 90% of people. Reduced need for medication.	Risk of death from surgery should be less than 1–3% in otherwise healthy people. Some memory loss possible after bypass surgery.	Approximately 50% of vein grafts are blocked within ten years. Internal mammary artery implant stays open longer.	If you want to avoid the discomfort and risk of open heart surgery, even though alternatives may have a higher failure rate.	*Medications:* nitrates, beta-blockers, calcium channel blockers. *Risk factor reduction:* reduced or modify elevated cholesterol, high blood pressure, smoking, sedentary life. *Other:* Supervised cardiac rehab exercise program. *Alternative procedure:* PTCA (balloon angioplasty-dilation of coronary artery). Other devices to remove plaque are in development.
	Unstable angina with one or more coronary arteries blocked.	Relief of angina, reduced risk of heart attack.				
	Significant blockage of the left main coronary artery (the blood vessel supplying most of the heart muscle).	Reduced risk of death and relief of pain if present.				
	Possible indication: multiple blockages in coronary arteries with symptoms easily controlled by medications.	Modest reduced risk of death and less need for medication.				
Cesarean section (removal of the fetus from the uterus by surgery)	Distress to the fetus during labor, infected vaginal canal (e.g., herpes), abnormality of the placenta (lining of the uterus), failure of labor to progress.	Prevents irreparable damage to the baby (and the mother).	Small risk from general or spinal anesthesia. Greater infection risk. Possible adhesions.	Caesarean section will prolong hospital stay.	If baby and mother are not threatened by normal vaginal birth.	*Medications:* trial of oxytocin infusion if appropriate.
	Possible indication: prior cesarean deliveries.	Prevents damage to possibly weakened uterus.				

Procedure	Indications	Benefits	Risks		When to consider alternatives	Alternatives / Medication
Dilatation and curettage (D&C—Removal of uterine lining tissue)	Diagnosis and treatment of abnormal uterine bleeding, especially after menopause. After incomplete abortion ("miscarriage"). To retrieve "lost" IUD. Insertion of radioactive implants	Thorough removal of bleeding tissue to stop bleeding and for pathologic analysis. Removal of remnant tissue. Cancer treatment.	Small risk from general anesthesia. Small risk of cervical tear or uterine perforation.		Women under 40 may consider alternatives, because cancer of the uterus is unlikely.	*Medication:* hormones may control abnormal bleeding. *Alternative procedures:* endometrial biopsy may be done in the office instead. Hysteroscopy may suffice.
Disc removal (for ruptured lumbar disc)	Ruptured disc (herniated or protruding and pressing on the nerves) with advancing symptoms due to nerve compression (for example, foot drop). Intractable pain not responding to bed rest and medication.	Prevents permanent nerve damage and loss of function. Greater than 90% relief of symptoms.	Small risk of vascular damage and nerve damage. Small risk from general anesthesia.		If one wishes to avoid major surgery with its inherent risk.	*Non procedural:* bed rest, weight loss, and traction. *Medication:* chemonucleolysis (dissolving the disc by injection) may be effective.
Hip replacement ("artificial" hip)	Intractable pain or loss of function due to arthritis or aseptic necrosis (loss of blood supply to the bone) that affects quality of life. *Possible indication:* inability to tolerate medication.	Restoration of function and relief of pain. Increased self-sufficiency and independence.	Small risk from general anesthesia, blood clots in the veins or lung, and infection of prosthesis.	Prosthesis (artificial hip) may crack or loosen in the future. Prosthesis may be cemented in or be cementless.	If function is not markedly impaired.	*Life-style:* weight loss, decrease weight bearing. *Medication:* nonsteroidal anti-inflammatory drugs (NSAIDs)

COMMON INVASIVE THERAPEUTIC PROCEDURES AND ALTERNATIVES (continued)

Procedure	Indications for Therapy	Expected Benefits	Risks	Special Considerations	When to Consider Alternatives	Alternatives
Hysterectomy (removal of the uterus)	Cancer of the pelvic organs.	Complete removal of cancerous tissue.	Small risk from anesthesia.	Less traumatic if it can be done vaginally (if there are no adhesions from prior pelvic surgery). If ovaries are removed, hormone replacement may be considered.	Not appropriate for birth control per se. If a woman wishes to have more children.	*Mechanical:* pessary may help in case of prolapse. *Medication:* hormonal therapy in women below age 40 may control excessive bleeding. *Surgical:* Myomectomy (removal of the fibroid alone) may preserve childbearing.
	Uncontrolled bleeding in a woman beyond childbearing years.	Removal of the bleeding source.				
	Symptomatic uterine prolapse (protrusion into the vagina).	Relief of discomfort.				
	Presence of extensive symptomatic (benign) fibroid tumors.	Relief of discomfort due to pelvic pressure and fullness.				
Mastectomy (removal of the breast)	Cancer of the breast	Removal of the entire breast cancer.	Small risk from anesthesia. May have arm-swelling after removal of lymph glands under the arm.	Some types of breast cancer may arise in more than one site in the breast. May have reconstruction after mastectomy.	If the tumor is less than 4 cm. (about 1½ in.).	*Surgical:* lumpectomy with removal of the lymph glands in the armpit, with follow-up radiation therapy. *Chemotherapy:* supplementary chemotherapy may be helpful.

Procedure						
Peripheral artery bypass (open up circulation in the legs)	Intractable leg or calf pain that significantly limits walking or other activity, and markedly affects quality of life. Threat of irreversible damage to the foot or leg due to lack of blood flow to the affected tissues.	Restoration of activity and life-style. Preserve the foot or limb and avoid gangrene and amputation.	Small risk from anesthesia. Risk of clotting in the blood vessel.	As long as the foot or leg is not threatened, the decision is based on function and comfort.	If one wishes to avoid major surgery with its inherent risks. For isolated blockage, angioplasty (opening up the artery) with balloon or laser.	*Life-style:* stop smoking, lower cholesterol, exercise. *Medication:* pentoxiphylline to lower blood viscosity. *Alternative procedure:* laser or balloon angioplasty.
Prostate resection (TURP) (removal of prostate tissue via the penis)	Restricted bladder-emptying causing symptoms of decrease in flow and incomplete emptying. Signs of kidney damage resulting from pressure backup due to blockage of bladder emptying.	Relief of symptoms and improvement of kidney function when applicable.	Impotence, retrograde ejaculation (backward into the bladder), bleeding.	Can be repeated if necessary. Open procedure (with abdominal incision) may be more effective.	As long as kidney function is not affected, and there is no suspicion of cancer, decision depends on symptoms alone.	*Medications:* may be available in the future to limit growth of prostate. Balloon dilation may be an alternative.
Vasectomy (cutting the tube that carries sperm)	A man's desire for permanent birth control.	Permanent birth control.	Transient bleeding or bruising. Rare possible failure to provide permanent contraception.	Essentially permanent birth control. Delayed onset of protection until remaining sperm are ejaculated. Easily done in office under local anesthetic. No effect on libido.	When there may be a desire to father children in the future. (Vasectomy can be successfully reversed sometimes.) When condoms are needed for infection control.	Condoms. "Male pill" may be available in future. Birth control for partner is an alternative.

COMMON INVASIVE THERAPEUTIC PROCEDURES AND ALTERNATIVES *(continued)*

FOUR INVASIVE THERAPEUTIC PROCEDURES

Procedure	Indications for Therapy	Expected Benefits	Risks	Special Considerations	When to Consider Alternatives	Alternatives
Arthroscopic meniscal repair (knee cartilage repair)	Symptoms caused by torn meniscus (knee cartilage): locking, catching, giving way of the knee.	Restoration of function.	Possible long-term risk of arthritis. Small risk from general anesthesia.	Rapid healing when done arthroscopically. May be repeated if needed.	If symptoms are not too severe and immobility and rehabilitation can be accommodated for 4–6 weeks.	Casting the leg for 4–6 weeks, followed by vigorous rehab program.
Laparoscopic tubal ligation ("tying" the fallopian tubes)	A woman's desire for permanent birth control.	Permanent birth control.	Small risk from general anesthesia. Possible failure (pregnancy).	Well tolerated outpatient "band-aid" surgery. No effect on libido.	When additional measures are needed for infection control. If future pregnancy planned.	Other forms of contraception: diaphragm, IUD, sponge, spermicide, birth control pills, or contraception for partner.
Colonoscopic polypectomy (polyp removal through the flexible scope)	Removal of polyp or biopsy of mass in the colon.	Removal of polyps and complete surveillance of the colon.	Small risk of perforation of the colon or bleeding.	Outpatient procedure with minimal sedation. Can be repeated.	Anytime a polyp or mass is suspected. Has essentially replaced surgery for this purpose.	*Surgery:* removal of a section of colon can be performed if colonoscopy is not sufficient.

Procedure	Indications	Effect	Risks	Comments	Cautions	Alternatives
Percutaneous transluminal coronary angioplasty (PTCA—opening a blocked artery to the heart with a balloon or other device)	When there is coronary artery disease severe enough to consider bypass surgery (see above). Possibly in the setting of an acute heart attack or several days after the dissolution of a clot causing a heart attack.	Can restore circulation to heart muscle fed by blocked arteries, relieving pain and increasing function. May limit heart damage in acute attack.	May cause spasm of the blood vessel. Rarely, may necessitate urgent bypass surgery.	Not for left main coronary artery blockage. Renarrowing in 25% of people in first 6 months. Procedure can be repeated. Helps 85–90% of patients.	Left main coronary artery blockage may be too risky for angioplasty. If multiple blockages are present, bypass surgery may be more appropriate if angioplasty has failed repeatedly.	*Medications and lifestyle:* See above on bypass surgery. *Surgery:* coronary artery bypass surgery.

THREE ALTERNATIVES TO SURGERY OR INVASIVE PROCEDURES

Procedure	Indications	Effect	Risks	Comments	Cautions	Alternatives
Chemotherapy (administration of medications for cancer treatment)	Treatment of malignancies that are not localized and cannot be removed. Adjuvant (supplemental) therapy after surgery and/or radiation.	Partial or total destruction of cancerous cells in all parts of the body. Prevention of late recurrence of cancer.	Medications may destroy normal tissue as well. Low resistance to infection, bleeding.	Some therapy protocols are in constant change and specialty oncology care is important.	When the treatment program for a particular cancer is not well established, consultation with surgeons and radiotherapists is advised.	Surgery, radiation therapy, immunotherapy, or alternate chemotherapy programs may all be helpful, depending on the clinical situation.

COMMON INVASIVE THERAPEUTIC PROCEDURES AND ALTERNATIVES (continued)

Procedure	Indications for Therapy	Expected Benefits	Risks	Special Considerations	When to Consider Alternatives	Alternatives
Radiation therapy (either by direct beam or with radioactive substances)	Treatment of malignancies that are localized but that cannot be removed surgically. Sometimes used as adjunctive therapy following or preceding surgery or chemotherapy.	Partial or complete destruction of cancer tissue, especially to relieve a localized blockage or involvement, such as in lung, bone, or brain.	May cause damage to the skin or to adjacent healthy tissue (e.g., rectum or esophagus).	Only some cancers are sensitive to radiation therapy. Skilled radiotherapist is important for best effect.	When the treatment program for a particular cancer is not well established, consultation with surgeons and oncologists is advised.	Surgery, chemotherapy, or immunotherapy may all be helpful, depending on the clinical situation.
Rehabilitation therapy (physical, occupational, or speech therapy)	After injury such as stroke or heart attack, after orthopedic surgery or injury. For functionally limited heart, lung, or arthritis patients.	Help restore function and independence if possible. Maximal development of existing strength and potential to compensate for weaknesses.	Injury due to overzealous participation.	Motivation is often a limiting factor. Personality of therapist may be a key to success. Rehab may allow a reduction of medications.		Rehabilitation therapy is always an adjunct to other therapy. Home self-directed program may replace formal therapy.

ASSESSING THE ALTERNATIVES FOR TREATMENT

Sometimes clear alternatives to surgery are evident on an "either-or" basis, but most often this is not the case and the matter is more complicated. Many cancer treatments, for example, include combinations of surgery, chemotherapy, and radiation therapy, depending on the stage of the disease and the condition of the patient. The efficacy of one treatment or another may change dramatically as the cancer advances or regresses. Similarly, for a patient with coronary artery disease, the choices between medications, angioplasty, and open-heart bypass surgery can change quickly as the patient's condition changes.

When you choose between one form of treatment and another, at any given time, it may not be enough to consider only the success rates of the various approaches. Remember the rule that every treatment involves costs that must be weighed against the benefits. A man with prostate cancer may be treated at different stages of the disease with surgery, medication, or radiation. The surgery may involve the removal of the testicles; medication with female hormones may produce breast tenderness and enlargement; and the radiation may result in chronic rectal inflammation, incontinence, and diarrhea. The decision to use one treatment rather than another may boil down to a decision about which adverse effects are the lesser of the evils.

Aside from medication and surgery, few other therapies are definitive or complete. As a result, finding treatment alternatives can be frustrating. You should begin the process by asking your primary-care doctor about alternatives. As well as offering an opinion, he or she may recommend particular specialists to consult. A more valuable resource for information may be the consultants you're already seeing. Most specialists who deal with particular diseases have contacts with networks of other specialists who deal with those diseases, and they can provide preliminary information.

Be aware that some drugs and procedures are highly experimental and have been approved by the FDA for use on a trial basis by a limited number of physicians. Occasionally, such experimental therapies receive a good deal of attention in the press, as with new treatments for

AIDS, for example. But often, they are little known, and information about them is difficult to find. Organizations like the American Cancer Society may help you find doctors or institutions that are involved in therapeutic trials for emerging treatments. Local support groups that are focused on specific medical problems sometimes know a good deal more about what is going on in that particular field than many of the physicians in the community. They may provide information about where to look for therapeutic alternatives, experimental or otherwise.

Keep in mind that your search for treatment alternatives may be limited by the practical realities of time, effort, and cost. Your insurance coverage may not pay for multiple consultations, especially if you're enrolled in an HMO, so review your insurance contract to clarify whether the company will cover the therapies you're considering. Many won't pay for therapies that they consider "experimental."

THE DECISION TO FORGO THERAPY

There are times when therapy may not be effective or may no longer be useful. If you find yourself suspecting that there may not be any reason either to begin treatment or to continue it, you have several decisions to make.

Futile Therapy

Since most of us have high expectations of medical technology and tend to be unrealistically optimistic about our own situations, it may be difficult for a patient to admit that therapy either will not be or is no longer effective. We have noted often here that patients expect doctors to do *something* to help them improve, and for doctors, this expectation alone can be difficult to ignore. So patients may continue with treatment that's futile, and doctors may continue to treat them.

You can make a realistic judgment about whether or not therapy is working only by defining the benefits and the costs of the treatment and by continually revising the probabilities for these benefits and costs.

The decision to stop therapy will probably have to come from you. Doctors tend to be reluctant to recommend that therapy be discontinued, because the acknowledgment that therapy is futile is likely to be perceived as an admission of failure or defeat. However, your doctor is apt to be candid in answering questions about whether he or she thinks continuing therapy will be worthwhile.

Questionable Treatments and Quackery

When people are desperate, when they are offered no hope by traditional medicine, or when they are suspicious of the medical establishment, they often turn to unorthodox treatments. While some experimental treatments may be approved by the FDA for therapeutic trials that are administered by reputable physicians, others may be questionable at best, and at worst outright quackery.

Both questionable therapy and medical charlatanism are common in the treatment of certain cancers, AIDS, and other conditions for which there may be no consistently effective treatments. Testimony taken at the 1984 hearings of the U.S. House Subcommittee on Health and Long-term Care indicated that $27 billion dollars a year was being spent on health frauds, ranging from worthless cancer treatments and arthritis cures to cytotoxic tests and hair analyses.

More than money may be at stake when people turn to such treatments. One study, reported in the *Annals of Internal Medicine* in the mid-1980s, found that a significant proportion of cancer patients used unorthodox therapies either in conjunction with or in place of conventionally accepted therapy. Most disturbing was the finding that one-third of those people who relied on unorthodox therapy alone had breast cancer or blood malignancies that could easily have been treated with some success by existing means. For people who can't be helped by conventional medicine, questionable or even fraudulent therapies may sustain hope, illusory as it may be. However, when people who *can* be helped by established techniques turn to such therapies, they may be giving up the opportunity to obtain meaningful treatment and attention in time to make a difference.

Medical studies can show us the odds and probabilities that a therapy will work, but it's impossible to demonstrate that a particular treatment will never bring a remission or a cure. Those who prey on desperate patients exploit all of their fears and all of the human quirks involved in our judging and misjudging probabilities (see chapter 3).

Many quacks wave the banner of consumerism, citing the *right* of patients to use therapies they want despite the recommendations of the medical establishment, which they often portray as sinister. If you are tempted to explore a highly controversial "alternative" treatment, do include your primary-care doctor and a specialist in the circle of those you consult with before doing so.

SUMMING IT ALL UP

Unless you're faced with an immediate threat to your life or your health, don't rush—or be rushed—into treatment. Consider getting additional opinions and consultations to open other possible ways of dealing with the problem, and be sure to consider all your options.

Every treatment choice in medicine is a trade-off. The patient, weighing costs and risks on the one hand and benefits (or damage control) on the other, must decide on the lesser of the possible evils. Although the doctor should offer information and even recommendations, it's the patient's perception of costs and benefits that should guide his or her decision.

In making a choice, you should consider four basic questions: Is the treatment needed? Are the results reversible? What are the risks, the costs, and the benefits? Are the benefits worth the costs?

There is no risk-free procedure, whether the treatment is the use of prescription drugs or major surgery. The key to effective decision-making at each step of the treatment is to know the options that are available and to choose those that offer the least painful trade-off in terms of costs, risks, and benefits.

You will be making choices at virtually every stage of medical treatment. Working from the most clearly reversible procedures and those that carry the most easily controllable risks—where such treatment choices are possible or reasonable, and useful—we suggest the following sequence of choices: watchful waiting and supportive care, followed by medication therapy, followed by surgery or invasive therapeutic techniques. Each has its own schedule of risks, costs, and benefits that should be considered on an individual basis. In addition, you'll have choices at each stage of the sequence, from deciding on the therapy, to choosing the doctor, to understanding the procedure, to taking precautions against unexpected and unwanted consequences, to deciding to forgo or discontinue treatment.

No matter how carefully you investigate treatment options and assess the medical advice you receive, it's you who will live with the results of accepting or rejecting the treatment. Be sure you understand as well as possible just what those results might be.

Final Choices,
Final Decisions

Not many years ago, people died "natural" deaths at home in the company of family, and without the life-prolonging equipment that is now used routinely to keep human beings alive. This country's development of the sophisticated technology that saves and prolongs human life has led to a paradoxical situation: the placement of critically ill people—mostly the elderly—into hospitals, where the capability to save lives often serves only to extend the dying process. If current trends continue, you are likely to die in a hospital or a nursing home, and at some point you may very well be connected to life-support systems.

For many people the decisions that govern the use of such systems and the decisions about the termination of life-sustaining treatment—for themselves or for loved ones—may be among the most important medical decisions of their lives. But unless you consider your options and prepare in advance, these decisions will be made by strangers, and the choices may not be the ones that you or your loved ones would have preferred.

THE CHANGING FACE OF DEATH

We humans are different from all other animals on this planet because we alone can have knowledge of our own mortality. As people get older, they become increasingly aware that they will die someday, but in the past there was little that could be done to influence the inevitable processes of aging, dying, and death itself. Until quite recently, there was little controversy about what conditions mark the precise difference between life and death, and the question of *when* death occurs was neither particularly important nor even relevant. During the last fifty years, however, the acceleration of medical discoveries has created vital new issues and new problems concerning illness, dying, and death.

The Increase in Life Expectancy

Over the centuries, while the maximum life span of humans has not increased beyond about 110 years, the *average* life span has been extended dramatically: from less than 20 years in ancient Greece to more than 70 years in the United States today. In this century alone, average American life expectancy has jumped from 47 to 75 years, and the most dramatic increases have occurred among the elderly. Once an average American man has reached the age of 65, he can expect to live another 15 years, and a typical American woman can expect to live 19 years beyond the age of 65. Moreover, the rate of life extension is accelerating rapidly. It is estimated that in the next 50 years, the number of elderly in the country will double and that Americans over 65 years of age will constitute more than 20 percent of the population. In fact, the fastest-growing age group is those who are 85 and older. This group of the "very old" is expected to triple in the next 50 years, from 2 million to 6 million people.

As a result of this aging trend, an increasing proportion of Americans are now facing, and will continue to face, the chronic diseases that cause a progressive decline in health and often a lingering dying. Fifty percent of cancer victims, for example, are over 65. For these Americans, dying is often an extended experience, prolonged by medical technology that sometimes provides the semblance of life at a high cost in physical pain, mental anguish, and money. A report in *The New England Journal of Medicine* in the mid 1980s estimated that nearly 80 percent of the medical expenses throughout a person's life will be spent in the last two or three months of that life.

What Is Death?

The haunting decision of when or whether to be kept alive by artificial life-support systems rests on a major question: When does death occur? The boundaries between life and death have become increasingly blurred in this high-technology age of medicine. The moment of irreversible death rarely coincides with the moment that the heart or the lungs stop functioning, and the brain may continue working for as long as 45 minutes after breathing has stopped, even when many of the nerve cells have been destroyed. In fact, procedures such as open-heart surgery are actually performed during a time when the patient has neither an independent heart function nor an independent respiratory function.

Today, it is generally agreed that the pumping of the heart and the expansion and contraction of the lungs operate mainly to keep the body organs functioning, but the part of the body that is most important in maintaining one's identity as a person is the brain. In some cases, when the part of the brain on which consciousness depends is irreversibly destroyed, the subcortical centers that control breathing and other basic body activities continue to function. Although different organs and tissues in the body die at different rates, the *Ethics Manual* of the American College of Physicians echoes the prevailing clinical, legal, and religious view that death occurs when the brain has died, even though some of the body functions may continue.

To the courts and the medical establishment, "clinical death" is still a purely biological concept. But other serious questions are involved in the matter, particularly the issue of personal integrity. While there may be general agreement on the definition of clinical death, there is no consensus on when dying people stop being "persons." Your own answer, of course, will depend largely on your individual perspective, your religious convictions, and your philosophy of life. Some people believe that clinical and biological functioning are the only signals that have meaning, and that these should be prolonged at any cost. Others think that the criterion should be the "quality of life," and that the person for whom this quality of life has become negative—the person who is permanently comatose, or the one for whom life has become intolerable—may already have died a cultural, if not a biological, death. Because there is no universal agreement on the definition of death, someone you don't even know, acting on assumptions with which you may strongly disagree, may make treatment decisions about your own life and death unless you make your own decisions early.

Doctors' Attitudes Toward Death

The basic emotions and reactions to death have not changed much in the last several thousand years. Men and women have always been fearful of death. Nevertheless, there have been dramatic changes in recent years in our attitudes toward both death and dying.

Dr. Elisabeth Kübler-Ross, a recognized authority on the issues of death and dying, observes that the advances of medicine have made the process of dying more lonely, more mechanical, and more de-humanized. As a result, while people are still terrified of death, many now are more afraid of the ways in which they are likely to die than of death itself.

To many of the very old and particularly the terminally ill, death may not necessarily be the enemy. Many patients, particularly those for whom dying has become an extended process, come to accept it as a welcome release from pain or depletion.

Most patients have had neither the personal experiences nor the training that would prepare them to deal with their own dying, and assume that physicians are far more at ease than they in confronting the mysteries they ascribe to the matter. Yet most physicians are specifically trained *not* to deal with death. As a result of their education and conditioning, most doctors believe their responsibility is to keep patients alive, and they are afraid of feeling helpless when dealing with sick people. Most are ill equipped to handle death, either as physicians or as bystanders, because they have not acquired the skills of helping patients deal with the experience of dying.

Some years ago, psychologist Herman Feifel and his colleagues presented to the American Psychological Association a study showing that among groups of physicians, seriously ill patients, and generally healthy individuals, the doctors were the most reluctant to discuss death. Doctors react to death in a variety of ways, but as a group, they have been trained to look upon the recovery, or even the survival, of a patient as a professional victory and the death of a patient as a defeat.

Because of their increasing recognition that physicians are not dealing adequately with the needs of dying patients, leaders in medical training have initiated changes in the curricula of schools of medicine and nursing. In the past decade or so, the teaching of medical ethics has become almost standard in American medical colleges, and these courses almost always include extended consideration of the treatment of the dying. While the value of medical ethics courses has still not been adequately assessed, a survey reported in the *Journal of the American Medical Association* in 1985 showed that those students who had taken such courses believed that they were helpful in making doctors more aware of the importance of "compassion" when dealing with their patients.

Even more important than attitudes, however, is medical *behavior* with regard to the dying, and this is an area that has been generally ignored in medical school curricula. Doctors may recognize the importance of compassion, but they are seldom taught the *techniques* of compassion, as they are taught techniques for dealing with cardiac arrest, for example. They are rarely, if ever, taught *how* to deal professionally with death, how to empathize and not merely to sympathize. They have not learned the value of comforting, the simple techniques of hand-holding and physical touching, or the art of writing condolence letters to families. As a result, doctors frequently consider such techniques of comforting extraneous to their practice of medicine, and they are often professionally, as well as personally, uncomfortable with dying patients or with the families of these patients. One study of physicians' attitudes toward death, reported in the *Archives of Internal Medicine*, found that "physicians have less personal contact with the family at the patient's death than had been previously believed," and that "less than 10 percent routinely initiated subsequent family contact." Schools of nursing are far more advanced in this area. Nurses are more frequently being trained in the behavior of comforting the dying, of easing the passage to death, and this behavior is increasingly manifested on the oncology floors of hospitals.

THE RIGHT TO BE INFORMED

The *Ethics Manual* of the American College of Physicians proclaims that all patients have the right to be informed of their medical condition, its prognosis, and the alternatives for treatment. According to legal statute, physicians must provide such information so that patients can make rational decisions to accept or reject diagnostic and treatment measures. However, all too often doctors and families deny patients information about the diagnosis of a terminal condition or impending death.

Certainly there are patients who want only to be reassured, who want to be shielded from the painful truth, even when they may suspect that they are dying. But many others—and studies in the last 25 years show that they are in the majority—want to know the truth.

Patients actually are less anxious when they are told the truth, and withholding the truth from them can cause them to feel confused and isolated. Many patients suspect that information is being withheld, and they infer more than is true. An article in *The New England Journal of Medicine* in April 1984, co-written by 10 prominent physicians, outlined a statement of the physician's responsibility toward hopelessly ill patients, and concluded that

> practically all patients, even disturbed ones, are better off knowing the truth. A decision not to tell the patient the truth because of fear of his or her emotional or psychological inability to handle such information is rarely if ever justified. . . . The anxiety of dealing with the unknown can be far more upsetting than the grief of dealing with a known, albeit tragic truth.

The physician's obligation to inform also implies a collateral responsibility to advise. Writing in the *American Journal of Medicine*, cardiologist Rodney Falk comments that when a patient can no longer benefit from prolonged treatment,

> physicians *are* justified in advising that further therapy is of no avail if the prognosis is clearly hopeless. . . . To consult with a family regarding termination of therapy should *not* mean placing the decision solely in their hands, as so often happens. This induces guilt that they have somehow brought about the premature death of their loved one.

It is the same sense of guilt that often motivates a dying patient's family to enter into a conspiracy of silence, largely because, like many physicians, they project their own fear of death onto the patient. This conspiracy of silence usually involves more than just the refusal to acknowledge that the patient is dying. It can mean that those surrounding the patient refuse to talk at all, except to offer transparently false reassurances. As a result, those who are isolated by the screen of silence may feel abandoned and helpless.

The abandonment can be quite literal. Physicians who are uncomfortable with the dying may write off a patient emotionally, cutting short or even eliminating their visits because they may believe that there is nothing more that they can do. As a result, their patients are denied choices even about their own deaths. These choices go far beyond the obvious decisions of the way and the place in which one chooses to die. Someone with terminal cancer, for example, may well choose to forgo painful or protracted treatments if he or she knows that the most that can be gained is a few months more of life, and may choose, instead, to prepare for a shorter but less painful life span. As long as survival is the only goal that doctors set, the uninformed patient is isolated and denied choices that may be at least as important as life itself.

Individual doctors vary as to how much information they want to give. Some tell patients as much as *they* think the patients need. Others, swept up in the new medical ethics and the philosophy of defensive medicine, are more open, some even going so far as to force information on patients who may not be able to cope with it. Still others try to determine how much information their patients want to hear.

For you, as a patient or as a family member or decision-maker for a dying patient, it is important to be able to guide the discussion so you can determine what is useful and necessary for your purposes.

First, consider your own personality needs. Decide how much information you want. Are you interested in general information? In details? In every contingency? Communicate your preferences to your doctor and your family.

Second, decide whether alertness or comfort is more important for you. Ask the doctor to explain the effects of various levels of sedation and pain medications, and even what to expect without sedation.

If you find that you just can't assimilate what the doctor is telling you at any time, feel free to ask the physician to return at a later time and meanwhile to write down the information so that you and your family can review it when you are emotionally more receptive. It may be useful to have other members of the family present during the doctor's explanation.

People are not being morbid if they discuss these issues early, although families and doctors often accuse them of giving up because they raise such end-of-life concerns. If you are seriously ill, knowing that you will be treated according to your desires can provide tremendous peace of mind and even free personal energy that would otherwise be used to struggle with family and medical personnel. Furthermore, once you have passed into the clearly dying stage, it may be too late to deal with these important questions. When people are dying, they are much too busy to think about death.

WITHHOLDING LIFE SUPPORT

There are two distinct types of life-and-death decisions that are often confused: the decision to initiate life-support measures — that is, the decision to "plug in," and the decision to stop life-sustaining treatment once it has begun — the decision to "pull the plug." Each issue has its own legal and ethical dimensions.

If you are in a hospital and your life is in the balance, you will be connected to life-sustaining machinery almost as a matter of course. You will not need to initiate the procedure. Conversely, you will usually need to do nothing in order to remain on the system for as long as it is needed to sustain life. The only issue will be your right to stay out of the system, or to get out of it once you're in, if you so choose.

The Right to Refuse Life-Prolonging Treatment

Two sets of legal principles may come into conflict when a patient refuses life-sustaining treatment: the right of the individual to privacy and the right of the state to protect and preserve life. Unless an innocent third party is involved, as in the case of a pregnant woman who faces a life-or-death decision, the courts will normally respect the individual's right to die of natural causes without intervening.

The right to refuse life-prolonging care is reserved for those who are deemed to be "competent" — that is, the patient is able to understand the consequences of choices and to make rational decisions. The right of the competent patient to decide has a corollary: the duty of the doctor to provide accurate information. In particular, the physician is obligated to supply patients or surrogates, to whom the patients have delegated the authority to make decisions for them, with information on the likely course of the illness if treatment is not given, the projected effectiveness of various treatments, and the price the patient is likely to pay for treatment in terms of discomfort, disability, and money.

When considering any life-prolonging treatment—medications, surgery, or even the administration of fluid and nutritional supplements—a patient or surrogate should ask:

- What will the treatment accomplish? What are the odds that it will work?
- What is likely to happen without treatment?
- What are the adverse effects of the treatment?
- If I refuse treatment now, can I change my mind later—and if I do, will the treatment be as effective?

The Right to Stay Dead

Strangely enough, even as the right to be allowed to die naturally is gaining wide recognition among physicians as well as jurists, the more fundamental right to remain dead—the right not to be brought back to life—is shrouded in ambiguities. Cardiopulmonary resuscitation (CPR) is different from other life-prolonging measures because once the need for CPR arises, patients are no longer capable of participating in the decision-making process, and they may never regain their decision-making capacity. Unless a patient has considered the possibility of CPR in advance, when he or she was clearly competent, and has specifically prohibited it, CPR will be administered routinely when body functions fail. Surrogate decision-makers are often required for subsequent CPR decisions.

Cardiopulmonary resuscitation was developed originally as a means for reviving victims of sudden cardiac or respiratory failure. For otherwise relatively healthy victims of electrical shock, drowning, drug reactions, heart attack, or a sudden complication during surgery, CPR is a way to prevent sudden death and restore the victims to functional life. Studies show that those recipients of CPR who had been functioning normally before the acute event were able to leave the hospital about 15 percent to 25 percent of the time.

The problem is that CPR has become a standard procedure for

attempting to revive any patient in the hospital, including the terminally ill. Very few such high-risk patients, including nursing-home patients, hospitalized patients with serious chronic medical illnesses, and the very old who suffered a cardiac arrest outside of the hospital, ever leave the hospital after receiving these procedures. In the groups studied, doctors were able to restore heart and lung function to these high-risk patients 30 percent to 60 percent of the time, but this "success" merely prolonged the hospital stay and delayed death in all but 4 percent or less of patients.

In 1983, the President's Commission on Ethical Problems in Medicine stated that "a competent and informed patient or an incompetent patient's surrogate is entitled to decide with the attending physician that an order against resuscitation should be written on the chart." However, the vast majority of patients in hospitals fail to indicate their wishes with regard to resuscitation. They may not have considered the possibility of CPR, or they may be reluctant to raise the subject. Currently, it is standard practice to attempt CPR on any patient who has a cardiac arrest in the hospital, regardless of the underlying illness, and on any patient outside the hospital for whom the emergency medical units are called.

In 1988, New York became the first state to develop extremely detailed statutes regarding CPR. The New York law mandates resuscitation for all hospital patients, even if they have terminal cancer, unless a competent patient decides against resuscitation orally or in writing, has a legally designated surrogate who can decide, or unless two physicians agree in writing that attempts at CPR would be medically futile.

Nevertheless, it isn't always possible, even in New York, to predict how the hospital staff will handle your case if you stop breathing, or if your heart stops. Dr. John La Puma of the University of Chicago Hospitals Section of Clinical Ethics and his colleagues surveyed faculty, intern, and resident physicians and found that the "do-not-resuscitate" (DNR) order was interpreted in different ways by different doctors. For example, 11 percent of the doctors indicated that they would still resuscitate by using chest compression (without the use of machinery) if a DNR patient suffered a cardiopulmonary arrest.

The Joint Commission on Accreditation of Hospitals in 1987 required each member hospital to establish standard policies governing resuscitation. These staff-developed policies must spell out how DNR decisions are to be made, how disputes are to be resolved, and how patients' rights are to be protected. The American Medical Association's Judicial Council has issued a number of statements which recognize that there are times when it is unnecessary, and even bad medicine, to resuscitate seriously ill patients.

Just as many patients fail to address the issue of resuscitation early enough, most physicians don't consider the issue until late in the course of hospital treatment, usually when their patients are so ill that death is imminent. In general, unless patients and their families take the initiative, the matter of whether or not to resuscitate probably won't come up until there is a crisis or until the procedure has already been initiated.

How to Decide About DNR

There are three basic questions to answer before asking a doctor to issue a DNR order for you or for a family member: Is the success of CPR so unlikely that the procedure would be futile? Is the patient's quality of life already intolerable? Would the patient's quality of life be unacceptable after a successful resuscitation?

The first question is a medical and technical one that requires a determination by the doctor. The problem is that many doctors are reluctant to admit defeat in advance, either for reasons of professional pride or because they worry about the reaction of patients' families. As a patient or family member, you can do little to influence the matter of professional image, but you can pose the question in such a way as to relieve the physician of his or her concern about the family's reaction. For example:

• Doctor, I know you're doing everything you can. But if my [or my father's] heart or lungs should stop, what is the real chance of recovery if you initiate resuscitation?

A good many physicians have expressed the belief that more patients for whom CPR would be futile would choose a DNR order if they were informed of the facts directly and clearly. Dr. Donald Murphy, writing about the problems in ascertaining the wishes of elderly patients at

Boston's Hebrew Rehabilitation Center for the Aged, notes that the issue is often clouded by the ways in which the staff communicates with patients. When patients were asked ambiguous or euphemistically worded questions like, "Would you want us to do everything possible to save your life if your heart stopped beating?" the usual response was positive. However, when information was provided that described the difference between a heart attack and a cardiac arrest, the nature of CPR and the ensuing intensive-care experience, and the approximate 3 percent who survived to leave the hospital, all but one of 24 patients decided against CPR.

The second and third questions, regarding quality of life, are value judgments that are within the patient's domain, and the judgment and the choice should be made by the patient or the surrogate decision-maker.

In considering all three questions, keep in mind that a DNR order means precisely, "Do not resuscitate." It has no bearing on any other treatment or options.

Choices May Be Limited by the Setting

A patient's choice to receive, or to refuse, life-prolonging treatment or resuscitation may be limited by the setting in which he or she spends the final days.

The home. When someone receives terminal care at home, the patient and the family have wide discretion to decide about life-prolonging nutrition and medications. Nevertheless, even if family members provide supportive services at home, a dying patient should be under the care of a doctor; medical personnel can provide more than purely medical attention, and can do much to ease pain and discomfort.

There is another very practical reason to have the patient under the care of a physician. Most states require that a law-enforcement agency be informed of a death that takes place outside of a medical facility. A death certificate signed by a physician who has provided or supervised care in the patient's last days can avoid the possibility of a full criminal investigation if there is any question about the circumstances of death.

You are under no obligation to call emergency services to resuscitate someone whose heart has stopped. However, once you do call, the paramedics who come with the ambulance are usually under standing orders to perform CPR. For a normally healthy person who has suffered a heart attack or an injury, this is appropriate treatment. But the family of a patient who is dying at home should consider in advance whether CPR would be an appropriate measure. Such planning would determine whether emergency services should be contacted, either by the family or by a caregiver or attending neighbor. It is common practice that once an ambulance arrives, the paramedics will begin resuscitation treatment, sometimes against the express wishes of the family or of the patient who has made his or her wishes known earlier.

A 1983 editorial in the *Journal of the American Medical Association* declared:

> We have wandered from treating sudden unexpected death to practicing universal resuscitation, and while universal treatment is unambiguous and avoids liability for failure to perform re-suscitation, it gives paramedics rigid and insensitive guidance for beginning resuscitation. Worst of all, it sometimes leads to inap-propriate and unwelcome intervention.

The best way to avoid this situation when caring for a dying patient is to decide on the procedure to follow in case of an emergency, and to make sure that caregivers are carefully instructed in how to act in a variety of situations. The doctor or home nurse, especially if a hospice organization is involved, can help you compile such a list of directions that covers:

- what to do for pain or agitation
- what to do for breathing distress
- what to do when breathing stops
- when to call and when not to call the rescue squad

The nursing home. State agencies have become extremely sensitive to the possible abuse or neglect of nursing-home residents, and many states now mandate both life support and resuscitation, in the absence of clear directives that indicate otherwise. In Florida, for example, the Department of Health and Human Services has decreed that all nursing-home residents must receive a minimum amount of nourishment and fluids, even if it is necessary to provide them by tube. In addition, if there is no advance directive to the contrary, many nursing homes require that CPR be instituted immediately and that the paramedics be called. The nursing staff or the attending physician may have little authority to withhold life-prolonging care or to prevent resuscitation unless firm instructions exist to the contrary, signed by the resident or a duly designated surrogate.

Ironically, a patient who is given CPR by paramedics called to the nursing home may very well have been under a DNR order when he or she was previously in an acute-care hospital. In fact, the personnel at the nursing home may be aware of prior DNR orders, but if they are required to call the paramedics, then the usual rescue efforts will be initiated.

Most nursing homes and long-term-care facilities encourage residents or their families to file an advance directive when they are admitted, in order to avoid unwanted rescue efforts. Regardless of the facility's policy, you should consider reviewing your options and writing and signing whatever directives you choose to supersede nursing-home policy on nutrition or CPR.

The acute-care hospital. In 1987 the Joint Commission on Accreditation of Hospitals required that all hospitals develop policies regarding the withholding of resuscitation efforts. As we stated previously, the state of New York has even passed legislation detailing how DNR orders will be implemented. But in many states the physician may have a greater range of freedom for writing DNR orders in the hospital than in nursing homes. Often, all that is required is to consult with the family and to document such a decision in the chart.

Remember that do-not-resuscitate decisions apply *only* to resuscitation and not to other life-prolonging treatments. For many insurers, especially Medicare, hospitalization in an acute-care hospital and the withholding of life-prolonging treatment (other than CPR) are mutually exclusive. Because Medicare will pay for acute-care hospitalization only when acute-care hospital services are needed and used, a decision to withhold life-prolonging care other than CPR will likely bring pressure from the Utilization Review Department to discharge or transfer the patient to a nursing home.

WITHDRAWAL OF LIFE SUPPORT

Some philosophers and jurists assert that there is little ethical, or even legal, distinction between withholding life-prolonging measures and withdrawing them once they have been initiated. Whether treatments are withheld or withdrawn, patients are denied interventions that may extend their lives and postpone their deaths. But from a practical point of view, there is a great deal of difference.

When judgments are made to withhold treatment, it is likely that the patient has been actively involved in making the choice. The judgment is made by the patient, the family or the surrogate, and the doctor on the basis of a prediction about the results of treatment or of inaction.

When decisions are made to stop a treatment, usually the intervention has *been shown* to be either ineffective or undesirable. Superficially, this factor would seem to make it easier to remove life support than to refuse it. However, in a large number of cases, the decision must be made on behalf of a patient who may be incompetent or otherwise unable to communicate his or her wishes, and the issue of the patient's desires may be open to question.

The Right to Disconnect

In 1975 the parents of Karen Ann Quinlan, a young New Jersey woman in an irreversible coma, succeeded in gaining court permission to have her respirator disconnected. Since that landmark case, the courts and the state legislatures have grappled with the issue of the rights of the dying to "death with dignity" versus the right of the state to keep dying people alive, even when there is clearly no hope of "cognitive or sapient life," the words used in the Quinlan case. The Quinlan decision was narrowly drawn and did not address the issue of withholding the use of nutrition and water, for example, as opposed to the mechanical devices that can keep people's body functions operating artificially.

Several other cases have helped to clarify at least some of the questions centering on the issue of denying food and water. In 1983 Paul E. Brophy, Sr., of Easton, Massachusetts, was diagnosed as being in a "chronic vegetative state" after suffering a stroke, but was kept "alive" for two years by zealous doctors and hospital administrators who would not accept his wife's pleas to disconnect the system by which he was fed. After the Massachusetts Supreme Court accepted the family's argument in 1986 and ordered the feeding tubes disconnected, Mrs. Brophy was presented with a staggering hospital bill for "treatment."

In 1982, in the case of 55-year-old Clarence Herbert, the California court of appeals ruled that physicians had no obligation to continue life support, including artificial feeding or hydration, "once it has become futile in the opinion of qualified medical personnel." This case marked a turn in the thinking of the courts. For the first time, an appellate court had equated the discontinuation of I.V. or tube feeding with the withdrawal of a respirator, a view that is gaining judicial acceptance.

Why Disagreements Arise

Surveys reveal that physicians and the general public alike have come to accept the idea of withdrawing life support to let a natural death occur if it is judged that treatment would only prolong dying. The results of the surveys also make it clear that the major reason for the disagreements that bring right-to-die cases to the courts is a failure among patients, their families, and their doctors to communicate clearly before the decision is made. A study reported in *Hospitals* magazine in 1987 showed that more than 80 percent of Americans would want life-support systems disconnected should they lapse into an irreversible coma. However, only 9 percent had prepared a written directive making these wishes clear. Another survey, reported in *American Medical News* in 1988, indicated that, while 56 percent of those polled said they had told their families their wishes about the removal of life-support systems, only 15 percent had actually signed a living will (see below).

The point was made even more forcefully in a poll of physicians conducted in 1988 for the American Medical Association. Seventy-eight percent of the physicians responding to that survey personally favored the withdrawal of life-support systems from the hopelessly ill if they or their families request it. The problem was that more than half of the doctors said that they were uncertain of the legal risks that might be involved in cases of life-support withdrawal.

The major reason for physicians' failures to accede to an advance directive to remove life-support systems is the fear on the part of hospital attorneys and some physicians that if the patient is permitted to die, the family will sue for failure to provide proper care. As of the time of this writing, no health-care provider has been punished or sanctioned for withholding or withdrawing treatment when that decision has been based on the patient's written directive or the concurrence of the next of kin.

Right-to-die cases keep coming to the courts, and the decisions in these cases mark the evolution of society's thinking about "pulling the plug." However, one should keep in mind that such cases arise only after the customary informal decision-making processes involving physician, patient, family, and hospital administrators have broken down. For the most part, when doctors, patients, and families communicate openly *and early* about options, right-to-die cases are highly unlikely to end up in court.

PATIENT'S ORDERS

The legislatures in virtually every state have enacted, or are considering enacting, statutes variously called "natural death," "death-with-dignity," and "right-to-die" laws. These statutes ensure that terminally ill patients have the right to direct in advance their own levels of life support by making declarations known as *living wills* or by designating surrogate decision-makers through a *durable power of attorney for health-care decisions*.

The Living Will

The specifics of right-to-die codes are described in legislative acts and court decisions, or "case law," which may vary considerably from state to state. While no two right-to-die codes are identical, they share many features.

All acknowledge the right of terminally ill adults to make their own life-and-death decisions through instructions to their physicians to withhold or withdraw life-sustaining procedures. These instructions generally are conveyed through a written and signed legal document called a *living will*. In all states, the validity of your living will requires that you prepare it in *advance* of the situation and at a time when you are competent, or of sound mind.

Legislation in every state that has enacted a right-to-die code provides immunity from prosecution or civil liability to physicians and other health professionals who act in accordance with the provisions of your living will declaration. Most of the laws specify that the declaration can be implemented only *after* your physician and one other doctor have certified that your condition is *terminal*. Legislators have taken pains to ensure that the living will not be an instrument for casual suicide. At the time of this writing, the law in two states—California and Oklahoma—provides that the living will is binding only if it is signed *after* a diagnosis of terminal illness has been made.

The various laws are quite specific in their definitions of life-sustaining procedures that may be included in the instructions, and some indicate conditions under which a living will is not operable. For example, in many states, living wills are not valid during any pregnancy; some are invalid if the fetus might develop to the point of birth; and others don't address pregnancy at all. Approximately half of the states categorically prohibit the withholding of fluids and foods, while other states leave that option open, to be decided as the need arises.

All of the laws permit the signer to change his or her mind. They provide for easy revocation of the declaration, in case you decide against it in the future. Moreover, your current wishes, written or verbal, supersede any provisions of your living will. This means that you are not locked into the commitment. However, to prevent the unintentional lapse of the living will, almost all states provide for the validity of the document unless it is specifically revoked.

Most of the state laws provide that if your physician is not willing to follow your instructions, he or she *must* arrange your transfer to a physician who will do so. All the laws specify that since a living will provides for a "natural death," the execution of a living will is *not* to be considered suicide, and that neither your life insurance nor your health insurance is therefore affected. In addition, most of the laws specify that nothing in the statutes is to be construed as condoning mercy killing. There are clearly stated penalties for forging or intentionally destroying a declaration or for concealing knowledge of its revocation.

If you prepare a living will, remember that it's your responsibility to bring it to the attention of your physician, who is then obligated to include it in your medical records and, in some cases, in the hospital charts if you should be hospitalized.

Most states provide a model form for the declaration. The major purpose of this model is to avoid ambiguous or confusing instructions. After all, such terms as "extraordinary" or "heroic" measures, which are often used in conversations about the right to die, are open to various interpretations if they are written in a living will, and the last thing you need at the moment of decision is a doctor who might think you meant something quite different from what you actually intended. In a few states, the form is to be followed *precisely and without deviation*. In most states, you have a right to add other specific instructions about what you want or don't want done. To avoid the invalidation of a living will by a poorly worded or questionable provision, such additions are considered *severable*, meaning that if they are found to be invalid or unenforceable, the rest of the declaration will still stand.

Samples of living wills are available. The one shown in this book has been included because it is short and explicit, and because it includes a proxy designation clause.

You should be careful to use a declaration that conforms with the law in your state, because there are some important state-to-state differences in definition. For example, the laws in some states do not include artificial feeding or hydration in their definitions of life support. If you live in one of these states and you don't wish to be kept alive by such means, you must take care to include the stipulation in your declaration.

In many communities, you can obtain a living-will form from the local medical society, from the social services department of a community hospital, or from a lawyer. If you have trouble finding a form, or if you prefer not to use local facilities, you can obtain a living-will form for your state at no cost by writing to: The Society for the Right to Die, 250 West 57th Street, New York, N.Y. 10107, or by calling the society at (212) 246–6973. If you live in a state that still doesn't have a right-to-die code, the society can provide a general model.

FLORIDA DECLARATION

Declaration made this _____ day of _____, 19____.

I, _____, willfully and
voluntarily make known my desire that my dying shall not be artificially
prolonged under the circumstances set forth below, and do hereby declare:

If at any time I should have a terminal condition and my attending physician
has determined that there can be no recovery from such condition and my death
is imminent, where the application of life-sustaining procedures would serve only
to artificially prolong the dying process, I direct that such procedures be withheld
or withdrawn, and that I be permitted to die naturally with only the
administration of medication or the performance of any medical procedure
deemed necessary to provide me with comfort care or to alleviate pain. I
do □ do not □ desire that nutrition and hydration (food and water) be provided
by gastric tube or intravenously if necessary.

In the absence of my ability to give directions regarding the use of such life-
prolonging procedures, it is my intention that this declaration shall be honored
by my family and physician as the final expression of my legal right to refuse
medical or surgical treatment and accept the consequences for such refusal.

I hereby designate _____ to serve as my
agent for the purpose of making medical treatment decisions for me. This power
of attorney shall remain effective in the event that I become incompetent or
otherwise unable to make such decisions for myself.

If I have been diagnosed as pregnant and that diagnosis is known to my
physician, this declaration shall have no force or effect during the course of my
pregnancy.

I understand the full import of this declaration and I am emotionally and
mentally competent to make this declaration.

_____
(Signed)

The declarant is known to me and I believe him or her to be of sound mind.

_____
(Witness)

_____
(Witness)

Making Sure the Living Will Is Honored

Simply preparing a living will may not guarantee that your wishes will be respected, and you should be certain to provide your doctor with a signed copy of the document, to be included in your medical records. It's best to make several copies of your living will so that you can give them to family or close friends, or to a hospital or another doctor should the need arise.

The best way to avoid overzealous or uninformed actions on the part of your physician or hospital staff is to be sure in advance that you and the doctor share an understanding of exactly what you want. Ask the doctor directly whether he or she is willing and able to respect your wishes, including any special instructions you may have added to the living will.

Since living wills can be quite general, if you have strong feelings about specific interventions and if you live in a state that permits additions, write them into the document and point them out to the doctor. The most common provisions deal with prohibitions against CPR and the initiation of mechanical ventilation and artificial nutrition. Think through some of the possibilities and specify your desires. If you don't want to be resuscitated under any circumstances, or if you want a DNR order to apply only when you become irreversibly comatose, write these specifications into the document. If there are any circumstances in which you absolutely would not want to be placed on a ventilator or be provided fluid and nourishment, then spell them out.

Even in states that have not enacted a statute giving legal recognition to living wills, the presence of such a document provides persuasive evidence of a patient's intention and carries great weight in court. However, it's useful to think of the living will as not simply a legal document, but also as a "memo for the record" to clarify your discussions with your family, friends, and doctors. Discuss the options and your preferences with your family so that there is no misunderstanding about what you want. Remember that the implementation of living wills does involve judgments about whether your condition is terminal with no hope for recovery. Don't assume that just because you have a relationship with a doctor, he or she knows what your wishes are about life-and-death decisions. For example, a study from Boston's Beth

Israel Hospital, reported in *The New England Journal of Medicine* in 1984, revealed that fully one-third of all patients who had received cardiopulmonary resuscitation said that they hadn't wanted to be revived, and that if they should have another cardiac arrest, they would not want to be resuscitated.

For reliable implementation of a living will, the issue of competence is critical. The courts have made it quite clear that competent patients have an absolute right to refuse medical care, even if such refusal results in certain death. Theoretically, the law presumes that you are competent unless it can be shown that you are not; but unfortunately, it doesn't always work that way. A physician may contend that a patient who has learned that he or she is terminally ill and is therefore depressed is not competent to make such a decision because of that depression. In the doctor's mind it is then permissible to ignore the patient's stated desires and push the family to seek an alternative program.

You can take several precautions against such circumvention of your wishes. First, prepare your living will while you are clearly *competent*. If you wait until you learn that you have an incurable or terminal condition, you may find it difficult to make a case for your competence. (Remember that in two states, California and Oklahoma, the document must be signed *after* a diagnosis of terminal condition has been made for it to be binding rather than advisory.) *Discuss openly* with your doctor and your family the subject of your death, and be sure that they understand your wishes. Such expressions of preference are often offered in court as evidence of your desires at a time when you yourself may not be able to communicate. By filing your living will with your doctor and with family members, you not only help protect its legal status, but you are enlisting allies who will help see to it that your wishes are obeyed at a time when you are unable to express or enforce them.

In those states that permit additions and changes, include in your living will a designation clause, authorizing someone to make decisions on your behalf if you should be comatose, incompetent, or otherwise mentally or physically incapable of communicating your wishes. Don't make assumptions. Be sure you discuss your desires with that person, and be sure that he or she is willing to act on your behalf as you would want.

Requests involving two areas of life support have been troublesome for those who have to interpret them: the prohibition of cardiopulmonary resuscitation for a patient suffering cardiac arrest and the injunction against artificially administering food and water to someone in a permanent vegetative state.

It may be helpful to check on the policy in your local hospital to be sure that DNR orders are permitted. You might also discuss with your own physician his or her position on DNR as well as the doctor's policy on noting such instructions in hospital orders, to be sure that nurses and other doctors are aware of their existence. If you and your doctor are in agreement on DNR, be sure that he or she notes this on the chart.

If you or one of your family members should be transferred to or admitted to a nursing home, be sure that a copy of the living will, with all appropriate additions and provisions, is on file there. Verify with the director or the chief nurse that the staff is prepared to adhere to its provisions. Clarify the conditions under which nursing-home personnel will call for emergency medical services, and if someone is under care at home, ask your doctor under what conditions your family should or should not call 911 or another emergency number. Make sure all your caregivers have this information.

The Durable Power of Attorney

Several states have specific provisions for naming a proxy or a surrogate—a person who is allowed to make decisions for you when you are incapacitated. The instrument for designating such a proxy is called a *durable power of attorney for health care.* A durable power of attorney is different from the general power of attorney, which gives someone the power to sell your house or buy stock for you. A general power of attorney terminates when you become incompetent through insanity or inability to make decisions for yourself, but this is just the time when you need someone to make sure that your decisions are carried out.

Although the word "attorney" is used, you can give a power of attorney to a family member, a friend, a minister, priest, or rabbi, or to anyone else you trust to make decisions on your behalf. While living wills apply only to clearly terminal conditions, the durable power of attorney for health care covers all situations when a person is unable to consider or make a decision. The surrogate decision-maker you have chosen, rather than hospital personnel or the courts, can resolve any ambiguities in your living will. In addition, the durable power of attorney gives the surrogate the authority to make decisions other than the implementation of the living will—to decide, for example, whether you should undergo medical tests when you are incompetent to make the decision yourself.

Like the living will, the durable power of attorney must be signed while you are competent, and in most states it must be notarized. One great advantage of the durable power of attorney is that it is recognized in every state and is likely to be honored throughout the country.

The durable power of attorney augments the living will by ensuring that the patient will have an agent to implement his or her wishes. Just as important, it helps resolve questions in the doctor's mind about the patient's wishes and relieves the doctor of concerns about legal responsibility if the patient's wishes are carried out.

On page 240 is a sample durable power of attorney, prepared by Barbara Mishkin and her colleagues for an information paper published jointly by the American Bar Association and the American College of Physicians, and distributed by the American Association of Retired Persons (AARP.)

Check the requirements of your own state by consulting an attorney or by obtaining a form from the social services department of a community hospital. You can also obtain up-to-date information about health-care powers of attorney and statutory forms for your state from either Concern for Dying or The Society for the Right to Die, both located at 250 West 57th Street, New York, N.Y. 10107.

WHO DECIDES WHEN THE PATIENT CAN'T?

Many health-care decisions, especially the choices made about life-prolonging treatment, involve patients who may not be in a position to make their own decisions. Patients may be incapacitated because of the illness itself, may have been incompetent to make judgments because of unrelated preexisting conditions, or may be minors. Each of these situations can create unique problems for making difficult medical choices.

[SAMPLE]*

DURABLE POWER OF ATTORNEY FOR HEALTH CARE

I, _____.
hereby appoint:

name

home address

home telephone number

work telephone number

as my agent to make health care decisions for me if and
when I am unable to make my own health care decisions. This gives my agent the power to consent to
giving, withholding or stopping any health care, treatment, service, or diagnostic procedure. My agent also
has the authority to talk with health care personnel,
get information, and sign forms necessary to carry out
those decisions.

If the person named as my agent is not available or is
unable to act as my agent, then I appoint the following
person(s) to serve in the order listed below:

1.
name

home address

home telephone number

work telephone number

2.
name

home address

home telephone number

work telephone number

By this document I intend to create a power of
attorney for health care which shall take effect upon
my incapacity to make my own health care decisions
and shall continue during that incapacity.

My agent shall make health care decisions as I direct
below or as I make known to him or her in some other
way.

(a) STATEMENT OF DESIRES CONCERNING
LIFE-PROLONGING CARE, TREATMENT, SERVICES,
AND PROCEDURES:

(b) SPECIAL PROVISIONS AND
LIMITATIONS:

**BY SIGNING HERE I INDICATE THAT I UN-
DERSTAND THE PURPOSE AND EFFECT OF
THIS DOCUMENT.**

I sign my name to this form on
_____ (date)
My current home address:

(You sign here)

*Check requirements of individual state statute.
Source: Barbara Mishkin, Hogan and Hartson.

WITNESSES

I declare that the person who signed or acknowledged this document is personally known to
me, that he/she signed or acknowledged this durable
power of attorney in my presence, and that he/she
appears to be of sound mind and under no duress,
fraud, or undue influence. I am not the person
appointed as agent by this document, nor am I the
patient's health care provider, or an employee of the
patient's health care provider.

First Witness
Signature:
Home Address:
Print Name:
Date:

Second Witness
Signature:
Home Address:
Print Name:
Date:
(AT LEAST ONE OF THE ABOVE WITNESSES MUST
ALSO SIGN THE FOLLOWING DECLARATION.)

I further declare that I am not related to the patient
by blood, marriage, or adoption, and, to the best of
my knowledge, I am not entitled to any part of his/her
estate under a will now existing or by operation
of law.
Signature:
Signature:

I further declare that I am not related to the patient
by blood, marriage, or adoption, and, to the best of
my knowledge, I am not entitled to any part of his/her
estate under a will now existing or by operation
of law.
Signature:
Signature:

When There Is an Existing Directive

Generally, certain conditions must be met for living wills and durable
powers of attorney to serve their purpose: The patient has to have been
competent, and the documents must have been drawn up according to
the appropriate statutes. In addition, the health-care institution and
the medical personnel must be aware of the advance directives, and all
parties must be willing to honor them. If all of these conditions are
satisfied, then decisions can be made legally and ethically on behalf of
an incapacitated patient without resorting to the courts.

When There Is No Advance Directive

Despite the publicity surrounding the right-to-die cases that reach the
courts, most decisions about dying are made privately and informally.
Physicians routinely turn to family members to make decisions to
withhold or withdraw treatment for patients who are incapable of

making their own choices. The law does support reliance on parents to make decisions for minor children, although parental decisions to withhold treatments may be overridden by the courts when medical personnel believe that it is in the best interest of the child to provide life-saving therapy. For practical purposes, when dealing with adult patients, medical personnel have virtually nothing to fear from withholding or terminating treatment as long as all the immediate family members consent.

Until recently, there was only one sure way for medical personnel to avoid civil or criminal liability when they relied on family members for instructions to withhold or withdraw life-sustaining treatment from incompetent or incapacitated patients: by going to court. The court would appoint a family member as the patient's legal guardian and delegate decision-making responsibility to that person, or sometimes the court would grant judicial approval for the decision itself. Fortunately, nearly one-third of the states have bypassed this potentially costly and cumbersome process by passing legislation that authorizes the families of adult patients to exercise the right of the patient to stop or forgo treatment without going to court. The statutes vary, but in general they require that if families are to exercise these rights, the patients must be incapable of making decisions for themselves and they must be terminally ill. However, some states allow such decisions to be made for patients who are irreversibly comatose. Several of the states prohibit the withholding of nutrition and fluids, and most of the legislation specifies the family members to be consulted.

Whether or not such provisions are in place, doctors and nurses still owe their first allegiance to act in the best interests of the patient. Obviously, directives from family members who are perceived to be acting in bad faith or out of ignorance must be rejected. But in the absence of explicit advance oral statements or directives drafted by the patient, neither family nor physician can be certain about what the patient would want done in a specific situation.

WHERE PEOPLE DIE: THE SETTING

Where people die is not always where they want to die. A survey of cancer patients in Connecticut revealed that while 67 percent of them had expressed a desire to die at home, only 20 percent of those who wanted to die at home subsequently did. When someone dies today, the odds are four to one that the death has occurred in a hospital or a nursing home, and for a person older than 65, the odds are even greater. Yet hospitals are not really designed to care for most dying patients, and nursing homes, for those who will never go home again, may be even more unsuitable. Unfortunately, the alternative of caring for a dying family member or friend at home is not always feasible, despite the best intentions of the caregivers.

Dying in the Hospital

Hospitals are busy facilities where patients are treated for such conditions as appendicitis, burns, hepatitis, operable cancer, and heart attacks. They are not designed as gentle refuges where dying patients can reasonably expect to obtain comfort, love, or an easy passing. Hospital physicians and nurses are trained to cure, to help people recover. They tend to be at their best when they deal with emergency and other acute care; they are not quite so good when they face situations in which they don't think their services will make much of a difference in a patient's condition, and are often at their worst when they deal with hopeless situations. This isn't because they are cold or uncaring. They simply tend to think in terms of treatment, and when they cannot provide meaningful treatment, many medical personnel feel inadequate. It is not unusual for many doctors and some nurses to be embarrassed, and even annoyed, when they face medical problems that call for comfort rather than treatment.

As a result, the dying patient is at the bottom of the hospital triage, the system of priorities for care based on a combination of need and chances for recovery. Dying patients are often the last to be visited by the doctor on rounds. Nurses are less inclined to answer calls from patients for whom they think they can do little, especially when they must direct their time and skills to those for whom they think their attentions will make a real difference. Except in oncology units and intensive-care units, the dying are likely to be ignored.

Even Medicare reimbursement policy reinforces the principle that hospitals are not geared for the treatment of the dying. There is no payment for terminal care as such in hospitals, and as a result, physicians must create a medical "need" to justify the admission of terminal patients for care. Doctors cite medical reasons such as "dehydration" and "intractable pain" so that they can order intravenous fluids or pain injections requiring the periodic assessment and discretion of a registered nurse. Ironically, these kinds of interventions may only add to the patient's problems by causing congestion from fluid overload, or disorientation or constipation from the side effects of the injections.

The most obvious reason why hospitals are not a good place to die is that they tend to be inflexible in meeting the special needs of dying patients. Operating rooms, intensive-care units, and even nursing units are conceived as settings in which medical personnel attempt to rescue sick people, to prevent death. Visitors are expected to stay out of the way, and they will be ordered out if their presence hinders medical efforts. But dying people require precisely the opposite kind of environment. This is the time for the family to be present, and it should be the duty of the hospital staff to stay out of their way.

No matter how carefully you plan, there is no way to be absolutely sure that you won't die in a hospital. There are particular circumstances in which a hospital may be the only reasonable place for a dying person, who may, for example, need to rely on medical technology to ease painful disorders that can cause additional severe suffering. Even in an "unfriendly" setting like a hospital, you can negotiate with your doctor and the hospital staff to obtain the best possible conditions for yourself or for a dying loved one (see chapter 5). This continuing exchange calls for the exercise of a degree of quiet assertion on your part—not aggression, because antagonism caused by a patient or his or her family is likely to arouse resentment and to be self-defeating—along with your expressed appreciation for the attentions of the hospital staff.

Dying in a Nursing Home

With the increasing proportion of Americans who live into old age, the number of nursing homes has mushroomed. By the end of 1986, about

1.4 million elderly Americans were in nursing homes, and experience has shown that about half of them never return home. For many such patients, the nursing homes provide little more than custodial care, and most custodial patients would rather be at home, especially when they are dying. However, unless there is a full-time caregiver in the home, such an arrangement isn't usually practical. Even if someone is at home, dying people may be deeply confused, crotchety, incontinent, or in pain. They tend to be a burden on the family, and their presence can greatly disrupt family life.

Particularly with the fragmentation of the family, typified by aged parents living in Florida or Arizona while the children remain in Pennsylvania or Ohio, a nursing home may be the only reasonable choice. Generally, nursing homes have become surrogates for the family in dealing with the care of elderly family members who can no longer care for themselves, whether or not they are terminally ill.

When a family member is admitted to a nursing home, it is important at that time to specify the treatment plans and goals. Under the best of conditions, the chances for successful CPR in a long-term-care facility or nursing home are dismal, and a living will is essential for specifying preferences about resuscitation and forced nutrition and hydration. If the family member is terminally ill at the time of admission to the nursing home, it is important to be realistic. Everyone involved in that person's care should anticipate that terminal care will occur in the nursing home without transfer to an acute-care hospital, unless the patient can't be kept comfortable with the resources in the nursing facility. Unfortunately, many families are unaware that Medicare covers only about 3 percent of nursing-home days, and that unless the patient is impoverished, little insurance coverage is available for terminal care in a nursing home. Medicare will cover rehabilitative services and certain arbitrarily designated skilled-nursing services, but supportive terminal care is usually not provided.

Only after virtually all of the patient's financial resources have been used up can the patient—or the family acting for the patient—apply for Medicaid. Some nursing homes accept only privately paying patients, while others will accept private payment, Medicare (when it applies), and Medicaid. Some are approved for CHAMPUS (Civilian Health and Medical Program of the Uniformed Services) or Veterans

Administration benefits. Still others will accept private funds and Medicare, but not Medicaid, while some will accept Medicaid only for those patients already admitted who have exhausted other funds and sources.

Since most nursing-home placements occur after hospitalization at an acute-care hospital, information about particular nursing homes is often best obtained from the social service and discharge planning professionals at the hospital. For more general information, you can write to the Nursing Home Information Service (NHIS), c/o the National Council of Senior Citizens, 925 15th Street N.W., Washington, D.C. 20005, call them at (202) 347–8000, or ask for information from the Peoples Medical Society, 14 E. Minor Street, Emmaus, Pa. 18049.

To register complaints about nursing homes, call the Nursing Home Ombudsman at this toll-free number: 1-800-342-0825.

Dying at Home

Less than a half-century ago, the vast majority of Americans died at home. There is much to be said for letting a dying person spend his or her last days in familiar surroundings in the presence of loved ones.

Unfortunately, many people underestimate the drain on the emotional resources of the family when a member dies at home. Dying at home may be neither as peaceful nor as humane as it has been pictured in Victorian novels or in romantic paintings. There is often a trade-off between the emotional comfort offered the patient who dies at home surrounded by his or her family, and the great pressure and strain on the family as it deals with the possible hemorrhaging, the multiple episodes of gasping for air, and the incontinence from which each family member is shielded when the loved one dies in a hospital or nursing home.

The gap between the vision and the reality of dying at home, and the realization by family members that they may not have the resources— emotional as well as technical—to care for a dying patient at home, may result in a transfer from home to hospital. According to a study reported in *The New England Journal of Medicine*, as many as one-third of those dying people who are cared for at home and who expect to die at home actually die in the hospital, even when they are under hospice care.

The financial strain, too, may be considerable. If a patient dies at home, the family can expect little financial support from insurance companies or from the government. Except for hospices, supported by Medicare, insurance companies tend to provide little in the way of home services for terminal care. Such home care, if it is required, is available from a number of sources: public tax-supported programs, community nonprofit organizations, and private profit-making firms. Each serves a purpose. Some of the public or nonprofit organizations require a physician's prescription or order for skilled nursing care, but not for custodial care. If you do pay for skilled nursing care offered by either public or private organizations, keep receipts and records, because such costs may be tax-deductible as medical expenses. You may include meals that you supply to the nurse or attendant, as well as additional amounts that you must pay for household expenses as a direct result of the attendant's services. For further information, send for *Medical and Dental Expenses*, IRS Publication 502, which is free of charge and available from your regional IRS center and some local IRS offices. This publication can also be ordered by using the toll-free number listed in your telephone directory.

The Hospice Option

A hospice, by definition, is a place of refuge for travelers. During the Middle Ages, the name was applied to homes for the poor or the sick. Modern hospices are places where the terminally ill are offered the comfort of dying in the company of their families and of caring professionals who are committed to "easing the passage."

Hospices may be institutions that offer homelike settings in which, unlike hospitals, the terminally ill can have visitors at any hour. In fact, in many of them a spouse, a child, or a friend is allowed to stay in the room to provide comfort for the dying person. A hospice may be affiliated with a hospital, although it will almost always be housed in a separate structure. It is likely to be staffed by psychologists, social workers, and counselors, along with medical professionals.

Hospice institutions may be no less expensive than hospitals, and like hospitals and nursing homes, their quality can vary considerably from place to place. With the growing popularity of the hospice movement, it is not surprising that some operators have come into the field primarily as a way to make money, and that some entrepreneurs convert or otherwise establish rooming houses that they advertise as hospices. Most states now provide for the certification of hospices just as they do for nursing homes, but state certification alone doesn't *guarantee* quality hospice care any more than it ensures quality nursing-home care.

Many communities have a hospice organization that does not provide physical facilities, but instead serves as an *outreach* program that offers services to dying people in their own homes. Such programs send visiting nurses to supervise home nursing care, as well as volunteers to provide practical help in the home and to help with the arrangements at the time of death. Where there are schools of nursing, student nurses may be assigned to visit or work with dying people in the hospice program.

Not all patients can qualify for hospice outreach services. A doctor must certify that the patient's estimated life span is six months or less, and there must be a responsible caregiver in the home to assume responsibility for the terminal care. For older patients, however, a major advantage of participating in a hospice outreach program is that Medicare then pays for necessary equipment, such as a hospital bed, as well as medication or oxygen required to provide the terminal care. As with on-site hospice facilities, the quality of outreach services can range from excellent to poor, depending in large part on the programs for volunteer training and supervision that are provided.

Some insurance organizations other than Medicare have begun to recognize that hospice care is becoming an accepted aspect of service for the dying. For example, Empire Blue Cross and Blue Shield of New York, one of the nation's largest carriers, has included in its hospital contracts coverage for up to 120 days of inpatient hospice care in a hospice or hospital. Also covered are home-care services offered by nurses and home health aides, social services, nutritional services, drugs and medications, and even bereavement counseling for the patient's family.

If you are interested in knowing more about hospices and in learning what qualities to look for in a hospice, write to The National Hospice

Organization, 1311A Dolly Madison Boulevard, McLean, Va. 22101, or call (703) 356-6770.

ACTIVE EUTHANASIA

"Mercy killing" and suicide are the most publicized of a group of acts known collectively as *euthanasia*—from the Greek word for "good death." The term is applied to all acts, both of commission and of omission, that are designed to shorten the dying process. However, most legal and medical authorities in the United States draw a sharp distinction between *passive euthanasia*—the term that is often applied to the right to die naturally—and *active euthanasia*, which involves an act of commission. Passive euthanasia includes such measures as the rejection of or withdrawal from life-support systems. Active euthanasia includes assisted suicide and mercy killing. Passive euthanasia rests on the right of an individual to self-determination and control over his or her own body, and to the right of privacy. Active euthanasia may place burdens and obligations, as well as possible guilt, on others. While the right to die by the withholding or withdrawing of life-prolonging treatments is widely accepted in this country, active euthanasia is a subject of fierce debate.

Mercy Killing and Assisted Suicide

Emily Gilbert, 73, was suffering from Alzheimer's disease, and her spine was disintegrating from osteoporosis. On March 4, 1985, her husband, Roswell Gilbert, 76, gave her a sedative, then shot her through the head. When he felt a heartbeat, he reloaded the gun and shot her again, this time fatally. That May, a Broward County, Florida, jury found him guilty of first-degree murder, and he was sentenced to 25 years in prison with no chance of parole. Jury foreman Sylvia Firestone told a *People* magazine reporter, "We gave him charity on the first shot. He was upset and overcome psychologically. But it was the second bullet that did it. That was premeditated." This comment underlines the legal distinction between a stress- or passion-driven homicide, which is usually treated as manslaughter, and deliberate mercy killing, which is legally regarded as murder.

Physicians, too, have been involved in mercy killings. Many members of the medical community were shocked in 1987 by the publication in the *Journal of the American Medical Association* of an article entitled "It's Over, Debbie." The article was an anonymous first-person account by a surgical resident physician who had administered a fatal injection of morphine to a young, terminally ill cancer patient suffering respiratory distress and obviously in great pain, after she had begged, "Let's get this over with." An Illinois grand jury subpoena, seeking the author's identity, was dismissed by Judge Richard Fitzgerald of the Cook County Circuit Court because of technicalities. The account itself resulted in an outpouring of divergent opinion, with numerous letters and editorials from physicians who either praised the *Journal of the American Medical Association* for opening a forum on a controversial issue or condemned the journal editors' actions as irresponsible.

A 1985 Lou Harris poll found that 61 percent of respondents surveyed believed that "the patient who is terminally ill, with no cure in sight, ought to have the right to tell his doctor to put him out of his misery." A 1988 poll of 600 physicians in California, published in the Chicago *Tribune* on April 21, 1988, found that 62 percent of the doctors polled approved of helping a person die.

In some parts of the world, such as the Netherlands, physicians are permitted to perform euthanasia for hopelessly ill patients after very strict and detailed criteria are met and a second, uninvolved, physician concurs. Since 1981, no Dutch doctor who has adhered to the stringent guidelines has been prosecuted. This contrasts with the United States, where mercy killing and aid-in-dying—supplying someone the means to commit suicide—are both considered murder, although, unlike the Florida jury in the Gilbert case, most juries are inclined to be understanding of motivation. Nevertheless, the fear of indictment and conviction makes both mercy killing and assisted suicide risky endeavors for both doctors and families.

Much of the discussion about the involvement of physicians in euthanasia revolves around *intent*: whether the goal is to accomplish the deliberate and direct dispatch of a dying person or whether death is incidental to attempts to provide relief from suffering. In this country, it is considered ethical and legal for a doctor to take aggressive measures to free a patient from pain, even if such treatment had the effect of hastening a patient's death, as long as the primary goal of the physician is to relieve suffering, and not to cause death.

Intent is difficult to ascertain, and the line between the relief of suffering and active euthanasia is hazy, even for the physician. It is generally assumed that some physicians, like the author of "It's Over, Debbie," knowingly administer *ad hoc* active euthanasia.

Many physicians, and most professional medical organizations, maintain that doctors should not participate in active euthanasia. The American Medical Association's bioethical opinions, while condoning withdrawing life supports in hopeless cases, assert categorically that the doctor "should not intentionally cause death." Others agree with Dr. Sidney Wanzer, a Concord, Massachusetts, physician who wrote in the American Geriatrics Society's *Clinical Report on Aging* that: "We are recognizing more and more that the welfare of the patient (the true goal of the physician) is often best served by death rather than life extension."

Whatever your own philosophy and preferences, recognize that the most effective way to approach the issue is to initiate open and frank discussions with your physician. Let your doctor know what actions you would expect, or hope, that he or she would take if you are ever in a position of hopeless suffering. Be sure, too, to anticipate the possibility that you may not always be competent to make decisions as an illness develops or advances. Discuss with your physician and with your family how you would want them to deal with specific situations such as intractable pain as an illness progresses. Patients' orders have meaning only if you plan ahead.

The "Self-Deliverance" Movement

In March 1983 the well-known novelist Arthur Koestler and his wife Cynthia were found dead in their London apartment, apparently the result of a deliberate overdose of barbiturates. Koestler, 77, who suffered from leukemia and Parkinson's disease, and his wife had been members of EXIT, a British organization dedicated to the right to "death with dignity." Koestler had once written in one of the society's pamphlets that, unlike animals, human beings do not expire "peacefully and without fuss in old age." In September 1988, 85-year-old

David Raff and his 87-year-old wife, Reba, each suffering from terminal illnesses, died in Sarasota, Florida, of self-induced drug overdoses. As members of the Suncoast Chapter of the Hemlock Society, their actions were praised by some members of the community, including fellow Hemlock Society members, but condemned by others as immoral.

These two cases bring into focus the issue of suicide as a means of avoiding or escaping suffering. The Koestler case was the subject of a sharp debate a month later at the annual meeting of the American Association of Suicidology, an organization of suicide prevention specialists, in Dallas. The focus of that conference was a newly published and highly controversial book, *Let Me Die Before I Wake*, by Derek Humphry, founder of the Hemlock Society. The book is described by Humphry and his associates as a guide for "self-deliverance" for the dying. Its critics view it as a suicide manual that may cause unnecessary deaths among the young and the depressed, people for whom the notion of suicide may be a temporary inclination that would pass were it not for the availability of a guide to self-destruction. Humphry draws a clear distinction between voluntary euthanasia and mercy killing, of which he disapproves. "The quintessence of voluntary euthanasia," he writes, "is personal choice and self control, with sometimes a little help from one's friends."

Some critics argue that the expression "rational suicide" is a contradiction in terms. Dr. Jack Willke, president of the National Right to Life Committee, contends that his organization cannot find any circumstance that would justify the violent taking of life. "We don't say that you have to use medication or mechanical equipment if the patient is in the process of dying," he says, "but one never directly kills." Dr. Willke believes that a physician who makes drugs available to a candidate for suicide is an accomplice to murder. A physician himself, he asserts that there is no such thing as pain that cannot be controlled. "If you can't control the pain," he observes, "get another doctor."

Religious leaders are divided on the issue. Some—perhaps most—contend that it is morally wrong to take one's life, that the decision must be left to God. Others, like John D. Arras, philosopher-in-residence at Montefiore Medical Center in New York City, think that God should be thought of as a compassionate innkeeper who gives his residents the right to check out whenever they like.

Not all of the right-to-die groups agree with the position of the Hemlock Society. The Society for the Right to Die, for example, which strongly supports the principle of passive euthanasia, refuses to make available do-it-yourself advice or instructions. Alice V. Mehling, the organization's executive director, says, "Suicide can be botched with rather unfortunate results." And A. J. Levison, executive director of Concern for Dying, says, "We completely support the principle of bodily self-determination. But the vast majority of people who want to commit suicide are depressed people who need counseling—and *not* instructions."

Keep in mind that while attempted suicide is no longer a crime in this country, assisting suicide is, and the physician or other person who aids in a suicide attempt is exposed to the possibility of criminal action.

If you are interested in more information, the following organizations offer a range of views, positions, and information.

The Hemlock Society
P.O. Box 66218
Los Angeles, CA 90066
Tel.: (213) 391–1871

National Right to Life
  Committee
419 7th St. N.W.
Washington, DC 20004

Society for the Right to Die
250 West 57th St.
New York, NY 10107

Concern for Dying
250 West 57th St.
New York, NY 10107

SUMMING IT ALL UP

Views of death and of the dying process have undergone radical changes in the last few decades. With increasing numbers of us living into old age, a dramatic increase has taken place in the incidence of the degenerative diseases that cause protracted dying. Sophisticated technologies designed to prolong life often prolong only the dying process, and the result has raised diverse questions about the ethics and the legalities involved in the decisions to extend or to revive life artificially.

The legal principles that have been evolving in this area have tended to grant dying people or their surrogates the right to make their own decisions about whether to extend life or to withhold or withdraw the measures that would do so. Many questions remain, however, about the conditions under which such decisions may be made, about precisely when they should be implemented, and about the definition of what constitutes artificial life support.

In an attempt to clarify and institutionalize the decision-making process, most states now allow the individual to prepare a living will to spell out in advance his or her wishes regarding life support. To be valid, the living will must be prepared in advance, according to the appropriate statutes, by someone who is competent at the time. One measure you can take to ensure that the living will is honored is to inform your doctor of its existence and obtain his or her agreement to abide by its provisions. In addition, you should apprise family members of the document and of its provisions. Certain areas of ambiguity may be clarified by your adding specific provisions to the model form that has been accepted in your particular state if such a statute is now in place there.

In addition, you can specify a proxy or surrogate to make decisions for you when you are incapacitated, by preparing a *durable power of attorney for health care.* This document is recognized in all states.

Questions of intent surround much of the controversy about the sanctity of life and the right to die, as their respective proponents describe them. Both the withholding and the withdrawal of life support are forms of passive euthanasia, which permits nature to take its course. Active euthanasia, in contrast, involves an act of commission, and is the subject of fierce debate in this country. Mercy killing and assisted suicide are the most publicized such forms of active euthanasia, and both are illegal in the United States. However, a growing "self-deliverance" movement has provided information to terminally ill individuals who consider suicide as a means of avoiding or escaping permanent suffering. Proponents of the right to "self-deliverance" have promoted the enactment of legislation to legalize "physician aid-in-dying" for those who request it.

The pattern of patients' decision-making in the area of death and dying is changing rapidly. The best advice that can be offered at this time, regardless of your preferences, is to plan ahead. Make your wishes clear to those who will implement your decisions, document them with a living will and a durable power of attorney, and communicate clearly with your doctor and family to ensure that your wishes will be carried out.

References

Abrams, F. "Withholding Treatment When Death Is Not Imminent." *Geriatrics*, 42 (1987): 77–84.

Allen, P. "Death Choice Lauded." Sarasota *Herald-Tribune*, September 21, 1988, 1B.

American College of Physicians Ethics Committee. "The American College of Physicians Ethics Manual. Part 1: History; The Patient; Other Physicians." *Annals of Internal Medicine* 111 (1989): 245–52.

———. "The American College of Physicians Ethics Manual. Part 2: The Physician and Society; Research; Life Sustaining Treatment; Other Issues." *Annals of Internal Medicine* 111 (1989): 327–35.

American Medical Association. *Bioethical Opinions of the Judicial Council of the American Medical Association.* Chicago: AMA, n.d.

———. *Current Opinions of the Judicial Council of the American Medical Association.* Chicago: AMA, 1981.

Anonymous. "It's Over, Debbie." *Journal of the American Medical Association* 259 (1988): 272.

Appelbaum, P., and Grisso, T. "Assessing Patients' Capacities to Consent to Treatment." *The New England Journal of Medicine* 319 (1988): 1635–38.

———, and Klein, J. "Therefore Choose Death?" *Commentary* 81, no. 4 (April 1986): 23–29.

Areen, J. "The Legal Status of Consent Obtained from Families of Adult Patients to Withhold or Withdraw Treatment." *Journal of the American Medical Association* 258 (1987): 229–53.

Aschoff, J. "Circadian Rhythms in Man and Their Implications." *Hospital Practice* 11, no. 5 (May 1976): 51–56.

Barnard, Christiaan. *Good Life, Good Death.* Englewood Cliffs, N.J.: Prentice-Hall, 1980.

Bar-On, Dan. "Professional Models Versus Patient Models in Rehabilitation After Heart Attack." *Human Relations* 39 (1986): 917–32.

Barry, M.; Mulley, A.; Fowler, F.; and Wennberg, J. "Watchful Waiting vs Immediate Transurethral Resection for Symptomatic Prostatism." *Journal of the American Medical Association* 259 (1988): 3010–17.

Beckman, Howard B., and Frankel, Richard M. "The Effect of Physician Behavior on the Collection of Data." *Annals of Internal Medicine* 101 (November 1984): 692–95.

Bergman, David. "The Clinical Gambler." *Emergency Decisions*, September 1988, 7–8.

Besdine, Richard W. "The Data Base of Geriatric Medicine." In *Health and Disease in Old Age*, edited by J. W. Rowe and R. W. Besdine. Boston: Little, Brown and Co., 1982.

Blackhall, L. "Must We Always Use CPR?" *The New England Journal of Medicine* 317 (1987): 1281–85.

Bogdanich, Walt. "False Negative: Medical Labs, Trusted as Largely Error-Free, Are Far from Infallible." *The Wall Street Journal*, February 2, 1987, 1.

———. "The Pap Smear Misses Much Cervical Cancer Through Labs' Errors." *The Wall Street Journal*, November 2, 1987, 1, 22.

Brecher, Edward M. "Opting for Suicide." *The New York Times Magazine*, March 18, 1979, 72ff.

Bresalier, R., and Kim, Y. "Malignant Neoplasms of the Large and Small Intestine." Chap. 81 in *Gastrointestinal Disease*, 4th ed. Ed. by M. Sleisenger and J. Fordtran. Philadelphia: W. B. Saunders Company, 1989, 1519–60.

Burns, R.; Graney, M.; and Nichols, L. "Prediction of In-Hospital Cardiopulmonary Arrest Outcome." *Archives of Internal Medicine* 149 (1989): 1318–21.

Bursztajn, H.; Feinbloom, R. I.; Hamm, R. M.; and Brodsky, A. *Medical Choices, Medical Chances*. New York: Delacorte/Seymour Lawrence, 1981.

CA—A Cancer Journal for Clinicians 37 (January/February 1987): 3–17.

Canterbury v. Spence, 464 F. 2d 772, 784 (D.C. Cir. 1972).

Carey, J., "The Faulty Promise of 'Living Wills.'" *U.S. News and World Report*, July 24, 1989, 63.

Casscells, W.; Schoenberger, A.; and Grayboys, T. "Interpretation by Physicians of Clinical Laboratory Results." *The New England Journal of Medicine*, 299 (1978): 999–1001.

Cassileth, B.; Lusk, E.; Strouse, T.; et al. "Contemporary Unorthodox Treatments in Cancer Medicine." *Annals of Internal Medicine* 101 (1984): 105–12.

Champlin, L. "Compassionate Withholding of Feeding: Are Physicians Protected?" *Geriatrics* 42 (1987): 37–42.

Charles, S. C., et al. "Sued and Nonsued Physicians." *Psychosomatics* 28, no. 9 (September 1987): 462–68.

Chassin, M.; Brook, R.; Park, R.; et al. "Variations in the Use of Medical and Surgical Services by the Medicare Population." *The New England Journal of Medicine* 314 (1986): 285–90.

"Chiropractors: Healers or Quacks?" *Consumer Reports* 40, no. 10 (October 1975): 606–10.

Cleary, P.; Barry, M.; Mayer, K.; et al. "Compulsory Premarital Screening for the Human Immunodeficiency Virus." *Journal of the American Medical Association* 258 (1987): 1757–62.

Colburn, Don. "Rewriting the Ethics of Life Support." Los Angeles *Times*. Washington *Post* News Service, April 8, 1986.

"Communication Can Reduce Prescription Misuse." *Geriatrics* 43 (1988): 21.

Connelly, J. "Informed Consent—A New Perspective." *Archives of Internal Medicine* 148 (1988): 1266–68.

———, and Campbell, C. "Patients Who Refuse Treatment in Medical Offices." *Archives of Internal Medicine* 147 (1987): 1829–33.

Cotton, P. "Confidentiality—A Sacred Trust Under Siege." *Medical World News*, March 27, 1989: 55–60.

Cousins, Norman. "The Physician as Communicator." *Journal of the American Medical Association* 248 (1982): 587–89.

Cramer, J.; Mattson, R.; Prevey, M.; Scheyer, R.; and Ouellette, V. "How Often Is Medication Taken as Prescribed?" *Journal of the American Medical Association* 261 (1989): 3273–77.

Danzon, P. M.; Manning, W. G., Jr.; and Marquis, M. S. "Factors Affecting Laboratory Test Use and Price." *Health Care Finance Review* 5 (1984): 23–32.

Davidson, Henry A. "Death by Choice—The Good and Evil of Euthanasia." In *Should Doctors Play God?*, edited by C. A. Frazier. Nashville: Broadman Press, 1971.

"Deliver Us, Lord: OBs Dwindling." *Medical Tribune*, November 10, 1988, 1, 12.

"The Doctor Isn't Talking, the Patient Isn't Asking." *Medical World News*, September 12, 1983, 47.

Doering, C. H., et al. "A Cycle of Plasma Testosterone in the Human Male." *Journal of Clinical Endocrinology and Metabolism* 40, no. 3 (March 1975): 492–500.

Eddy, David M. "Probabilistic Reasoning in Clinical Medicine." Chap. 18 in *Judgment Under Uncertainty: Heuristics and Biases*. Edited by D. Kahneman, P. Slovic, and A. Tversky. Cambridge, England: Cambridge University Press, 1982, 249–67.

Eisenberg, J. M., and Nicklin, D. "Use of Diagnostic Services by Physicians in Community Practice." *Medical Care* 19 (1981): 297–309.

Elliot, Neil. *The Gods of Life*. New York: Macmillan, 1974.

Elstein, Arthur S.; Shulman, Lee S.; and Sprafka, Sarah A. *Medical Problem Solving: An Analysis of Clinical Reasoning*. Cambridge: Harvard University Press, 1978.

"Failure to Take Medication Properly Problem in Half of All Patients." *Internal Medicine News* 18 (January 1984): 1.

Falk, Rodney H. "The Death of Death with Dignity." *American Journal of Medicine* 77 (1984): 775–76.

Feifel, Herman, et al. "Physicians Consider Death." *Proceedings*. American Psychological Association, 1967, 201.

Felch, William C. "Let's Make Medical Care More Accessible." *The Internist* 30 (August 1989): 25–26.

———. "The Uncertainty Factor in Medical Care." *The Internist* 27 (January 1986): 6–10.

Feldstein, P. J.; Wickizer, T. M.; and Wheeler, J. R. C. "The Effects of Utilization Review Programs on Health Care Use and Expenditures." *The New England Journal of Medicine* 318 (1988): 1310–14.

Fensterheim, H., and Baer, J. *Don't Say Yes When You Want to Say No*. New York: Dell Publishing Co., 1975.

Fischoff, Baruch. "For Those Condemned to Study the Past: Reflections on Historical Judgment." In *New Directions for Methodology of*

Behavioral Science: Fallible Judgment in Behavioral Research. Edited by R. A. Shweder and D. W. Fiske. San Francisco: Jossey-Bass, 1980.

Fisher, B.; Bauer, M.; Margolese, R.; et al. "Five-Year Results of a Randomized Clinical Trial Comparing Total Mastectomy and Segmental Mastectomy with or Without Radiation in the Treatment of Breast Cancer." *The New England Journal of Medicine* 312 (1985): 665–81.

Fisher, R., and Ury, W. *Getting to Yes*. Middlesex, England: Penguin Books, Ltd., 1983.

Fowler, F.; Wennberg, J.; Timothy, R.; et al. "Symptom Status and Quality of Life Following Prostatectomy." *Journal of the American Medical Association* 259 (1988): 3018–22.

Fuerst, M. "The Promotion Has Gone High-Tech; The Results Haven't." *Medical World News*, May 11, 1987, 34–53.

Gallivan, M. "Physician Offices Invade Clinical Laboratory Market." *Hospitals* 59, no. 20 (1985): 84ff.

Ghitelman, David. "The Natural History of Malpractice." *MD*, April 1987, 59–81.

Gianelli, D. "Many MDs Sued More Than Once." *American Medical News*, May 8, 1987, 2, 81.

Gibson, J. "Medical Guardianship Programs: When Strangers Must Decide." *Medical Ethics* 4 (January 1989): 1.

Goyert, G.; Bottoms, S.; Treadwell, M.; and Nehra, P. "The Physician Factor in Cesarian Birth Rates." *The New England Journal of Medicine* 320 (1989): 706–9.

Graboys, T.; Headley, A.; Lown, B.; et al. "Results of a Second-Opinion Program for Coronary Artery Bypass Graft Surgery." *Journal of the American Medical Association* 258 (1987): 1611–14.

Graf, B.; Docter, T.; and Clancy, W. "Arthroscopic Meniscal Repair." *Clinics in Sports Medicine* 6, no. 3 (1987): 525–36.

Gramelspacher, G.; Singer, P.; and Siegler, M. "Is Active Euthanasia Ever Justified?" *Clinical Report on Aging* 2, no. 5 (1988): 1.

Greene, L. "Transurethral Surgery." Chap. 78 in *Campbell's Urology*. Edited by P. Walsh, R. Gittes, A. Perlmutter, and T. Stamey. Philadelphia: W. B. Saunders & Co., 1986, 2815–45.

Greenspan, A.; Kay, H.; Berger, B.; et al. "Incidence of Unwarranted Implantation of Permanent Cardiac Pacemakers in a Large Medical

Population." *The New England Journal of Medicine* 318 (1988): 158–63.

Halberg, Franz. "Implications of Biologic Rhythms for Clinical Practice." *Hospital Practice* 12, no. 1 (January 1977): 139–49.

Hannan, E.; O'Donnell, M.; Kilburn, H.; et al. "Investigation of the Relationship Between Volume and Mortality for Surgical Procedures Performed in New York State Hospitals." *Journal of the American Medical Association* 262 (1989): 503–10.

Harris, Jeffrey E. "Defensive Medicine: It Costs, but Does It Work?" *Journal of the American Medical Association* 257 (1987): 2801–2.

Harty-Golder, B. "Informed Refusal." *Sarasota County Medical Society Topics*, July 1989, 2.

Haynes, Bruce E., and Nieman, James T. "Letting Go: DNR Orders in Prehospital Care," editorial, *Journal of the American Medical Association* 254 (1985): 532.

Health and Policy Committee, American College of Physicians. "Improving Medical Education in Therapeutics." *Annals of Internal Medicine* 108 (1988): 145–47.

Henry, K.; Maki, M.; and Crossley, K. "Analysis of the Use of HIV Antibody Testing in a Minnesota Hospital." *Journal of the American Medical Association* 259 (1988): 229–32.

Hilgers, R. "Myomectomy." Chap. 58 in *Gynecology and Obstetrics* 1. Edited by J. Sciarra and W. Droegemueller. Philadelphia: J. B. Lippincott Co., 1989, 1–9.

———. "Total Abdominal Hysterectomy and Bilateral Salpingo Oophorectomy." Chap. 57 in *Gynecology and Obstetrics* 1. Edited by J. Sciarra and W. Droegemueller. Philadelphia: J. B. Lippincott Co., 1989, 1–15.

Hillman, A. L. "Financial Incentives for Physicians in HMOs: Is There a Conflict of Interest?" *The New England Journal of Medicine* 317 (1987): 1743–48.

Himmelstein, D. U.; Wollhandler, S.; Harnly, M.; et al. "Patient Transfers: Medical Practice Triage." *American Journal of Public Health* 74 (1984): 494–97.

Holzman, David. "Body Sets Times for Taking Drugs." *Insight* (September 14, 1987): 54–55.

———. "Operate or Not? The Answers Vary." *Insight* (March 9, 1987): 55–56.

Howards, J. "Surgery of the Scrotum and Its Contents." Chap. 84 in *Campbell's Urology.* Edited by P. Walsh, R. Gittes, A. Perlmutter, and T. Stamey. Philadelphia: W. B. Saunders & Co., 1986, 2955–75.

Hulka, J. "Dilation and Curettage." Chap. 54 in *Gynecology and Obstetrics* 1. Edited by J. Sciarra and W. Droegemueller. Philadelphia: J. B. Lippincott Co., 1989, 1–11.

Humphry, Derek. *Let Me Die Before I Wake.* Los Angeles: The Hemlock Society, 1984.

Hunt, M. "Patients' Rights." *The New York Times Magazine,* March 5, 1989, 55–56.

Huttmann, Barbara. *The Patient's Advocate: The Complete Handbook of Patient's Rights.* New York: Viking Press, 1981.

Iezzoni, Lisa I. "Changes in Payment Policies: Impact on Physicians' Office Testing." *Medical Clinics of North America* 71, no. 4 (July 1987), 751–62.

Ingram, B.; Keifetz, N.; and Watkins, T. "A Stark Look at DNR by the Book." *Medical Tribune* 30 (1989): 1.

Isaacs, J. "Vaginal Hysterectomy." Chap. 59 in *Gynecology and Obstetrics* 1. Edited by J. Sciarra and W. Droegemueller. Philadelphia: J. B. Lippincott Co., 1989, 1–11.

Jachuck, S. J.; Brierly, H.; Jachuck, S.; and Willcox, P. M. "The Effect of Hypotensive Drugs on the Quality of Life." *Journal of the Royal College of General Practitioners* 32 (1982): 103–5.

Jemmott, John, Jr. "Judging Health Status: Effects of Perceived Prevalence and Personal Relevance." *Journal of Personality and Social Psychology* 50, no. 5 (1986): 899–905.

Joint National Committee on the Detection, Evaluation, and Treatment of High Blood Pressure. *The 1988 Report of The Joint National Committee on the Detection, Evaluation, and Treatment of High Blood Pressure.* NIH Publication no. 88-1088, May 1988.

Kahneman, D., and Tversky, A. "Subjective Probability: A Judgment of Representativeness." Chap. 3 in *Judgment Under Uncertainty: Heuristics and Biases.* Edited by D. Kahneman, P. Slovic and A. Tversky. Cambridge: Cambridge University Press, 1982, 32–47.

Katz, Sidney, et al. "Active Life Expectancy." *The New England Journal of Medicine* 309 (1983): 1218–24.

Kübler-Ross, Elisabeth. *Death: The Final Stage of Growth.* Englewood Cliffs, N.J.: Prentice-Hall, 1975.

———. *On Death and Dying.* New York: Macmillan, 1976.

———. *Questions and Answers on Death and Dying.* New York: Macmillan, 1974.

Lantos, J.; Miles, S.; Silverstein, M.; and Stocking, C. "Survival After Cardiopulmonary Resuscitation in Babies of Very Low Birth Weight. Is CPR Futile Therapy?" *The New England Journal of Medicine* 318 (1988): 91–95.

LaPuma, J.; Silverstein, M.; Stocking, C.; Poland, D.; and Siegler, M. "Life-Sustaining Treatment: A Prospective Study of Patients with DNR Orders in a Teaching Hospital." *Archives of Internal Medicine* 148 (1988): 2193–98.

Lazare, A. "Shame and Humiliation in the Medical Encounter." *Archives of Internal Medicine* 147 (1987): 1653–58.

Lee, Richard V. " 'It's Better to be Smart than Dumb' or The Clinical Importance of Ignorance." *American Journal of Medicine* 79 (November 1985): 548–51.

Leventhal, H.; Glynn, K.; and Fleming, R. "Is the Smoking Decision an 'Informed Choice'? Effect of Smoking Risk Factors on Smoking Beliefs." *Journal of the American Medical Association* 257 (1987): 3373–76.

Lidz, C.; Appelbaum, P.; and Meisel, A. "Two Models of Implementing Informed Consent." *Archives of Internal Medicine* 148 (1988): 1385–89.

Lion, J.; Malbon, A.; Henderson, M.; et al. "A Comparison of Hospital Outpatient Departments and Private Practice." *Health Care Finance Review* 6 (1985): 69–81.

Lipkin, Mack. "The Medical Interview: A Core Curriculum for Residencies in Internal Medicine." *Annals of Internal Medicine* 100 (1984): 277–84.

———. "The Medical Interview and Related Skills." In *Office Practice of Medicine*, 2d ed., edited by W. Branch. Philadelphia: W. B. Saunders & Co., 1987, 1287–1306.

Little, W.; Constantinescu, M.; Applegate, R.; et al. "Can Coronary Angiography Predict the Site of a Subsequent Myocardial Infarction in Patients with Mild-to-Moderate Coronary Artery Disease?" *Circulation* 78 (1988): 1157–66.

Macklin, R. "Who Should Make the Decisions When the Patient Can't?" *Medical Ethics for the Physician* 3 (1988): 1ff.

"Malpractice Insurance Cost Rises to $3.4 Billion." *Internal Medicine News*, January 1–14, 1987, 48.

McIntyre, Lynne. "Why Take the Fun Out of Medical Writing?" *American Medical Writers Association Journal* 2, no. 1 (March 1987): 2–4.

McKean, Kevin. "Decisions, Decisions, Decisions." *Discover* 6, no. 6 (June 1985): 22–31.

"MD's Risk of Right-to-Die Lawsuit Is 'Extremely Low.'" *Internal Medicine News*, June 15–30, 1989, 3.

Miles, S., and Crimmins, T. "Orders to Limit Emergency Treatment for an Ambulance Service in a Large Metropolitan Area." *Journal of the American Medical Association* 254 (1985): 525–27.

Miller, Roger W. "Doctors, Patients Don't Communicate." *FDA Consumer*, July/August 1983, 6–7.

"Misdiagnosis Sparks Suits." *Medical Tribune*, September 17, 1986, 5.

Mishkin, B. *A Matter of Choice: Planning for Health Care Decisions.* Washington, D.C.: American Association of Retired Persons Special Projects Section, 1986.

Morrison, J., and Wiser, W. "Cesarian Birth: Surgical Techniques." Chap. 83 in *Gynecology and Obstetrics* 2. Edited by J. Sciarra and P. Dilts. Philadelphia: J. B. Lippincott Co., 1989, 1–21.

Moser, M. "Cost Containment in the Management of Hypertension." *Annals of Internal Medicine* 107 (1987): 107–8.

"Most MD's Favor Withdrawal of Life Support—Survey." *American Medical News*, June 3, 1988, 9.

Mulley, A., and Eagle, K. "What Is Appropriate Care?" *Journal of the American Medical Association* 260 (1988): 540–41.

Murphy, D.; Murray, A.; Robinson, B.; and Campion, E. "Outcomes of Cardiac Resuscitation in the Elderly." *Annals of Internal Medicine* 111 (1989): 199–205.

Murphy, Donald. "Do-Not-Resuscitate Orders. Time for Reappraisal in Long-Term-Care Institutions." *Journal of the American Medical Association* 260 (1988): 2098–2101.

Natanson v. Kline, 350 P. 2d 1093 (Kan. 1960). Cited in Katz, J. *The Silent World of Doctor and Patient.* New York: The Free Press, 1984, 65–66.

Nesbitt, R.; Borgida, E.; Crandall, R.; and Reed, H. "Popular Induction: Information Is Not Necessarily Informative." Chap. 7 in

Judgment Under Uncertainty: Heuristics and Biases. Edited by D. Kahneman, P. Slovic, and A. Tversky. Cambridge: Cambridge University Press, 1982, 102–16.

The New York Times, February 17, 1985, section 4, 5.

Novack, D. H.; Detering, B. J.; Arnold, R.; Forrow, L.; Ladinsky, M.; and Pessullo, J. C. "Physicians' Attitudes Toward Using Deception to Resolve Difficult Ethical Problems." *Journal of the American Medical Association* 261, no. 20 (May 26, 1989): 2980–85.

Pappas, Nancy. "Technology Assessment: Cost, Quality Face Off Again." *Medical World News,* June 8, 1987, 64–81.

Park, R.; Fink, A.; Brook, R.; et al. "Physician Ratings of Appropriate Indications for Six Medical and Surgical Procedures." *American Journal of Public Health* 76, no. 7 (1986): 766–72.

Parsons, Talcott. *The Social System.* Glencoe, Ill.: Free Press, 1951.

"Patient Care: A Duty of Both Physician and Patient." *Medical Malpractice Review* 4, no. 2 (1987): 2–3.

Payer, Lynn. *Medicine and Culture: Varieties of Treatment in the United States, England, West Germany, and France.* New York: Henry Holt, 1988.

Pegels, C. Carl. *Health Care and the Elderly.* Rockville, Md.: Aspen Systems Corporation, 1980.

Pellegrino, E.; Hart, R.; Henderson, S.; et al. "Relevance and Utility of Courses in Medical Ethics." *Journal of the American Medical Association* 253 (1985): 49–53.

Polesky, H. F. "Update: Serologic Testing for Antibody to Human Immunodeficiency Virus." *Morbidity and Mortality Weekly Report* 36, no. 52 (1988), 833–40.

Pollner, F. "Coalition Fights Substituting Drugs Without Physician OK." *Medical World News,* April 10, 1989, 10ff.

President's Commission for the Study of Ethical Problems in Medicine and Biomedical and Behavioral Research. *Deciding to Forgo Life-Sustaining Treatment: Ethical, Medical, and Legal Issues in Treatment Decisions.* Washington, D.C., GPO, 1983.

Preston, Thomas A. "Do Physicians Twist the Maxim Into 'Secundum Non Nocere'?" *Medical World News,* April 13, 1987, 26.

"Preventing Shame in MD-Patient Contacts." *Medical World News,* December 28, 1987, 34.

Prout, Deborah M. "Policy Makers Discover Dr. Wennberg's Research, Foreshadowing the End of Laissez-Faire Medicine." *American College of Physicians Observer*, November 1985, 15–16.

"Public Supports Transplants, but Who Should Pay?" *Hospitals*, September 5, 1987, 86.

"Pulling the Plug: An Easy Decision Only for Yourself?" *Medical Economics*, April 27, 1987, 13.

Reade, J., and Ratzan, R. "Yellow Professionalism. Advertising by Physicians in the Yellow Pages." *The New England Journal of Medicine* 316, no. 21 (1987): 1315–19.

Reynolds, Roger A.; Rizzo, John A.; and Gonzales, Martin L. "The Cost of Medical Professional Liability." *Journal of the American Medical Association* 257 (1987): 2776–82.

Richter, Curt P. *Biological Clocks in Medicine and Psychiatry*. Springfield, Ill.: Charles C. Thomas, 1965.

Richton-Hewett, S.; Foster, E.; and Apstein, C. "Medical and Economic Consequences of a Blinded Oral Anticoagulant Brand Change at a Municipal Hospital." *Archives of Internal Medicine* 148 (1988): 806–8.

Ricks, T. "New Corporate Program Lets Employees Compare Local Doctors' Fees and Training." *The Wall Street Journal*, August 4, 1987, B1.

"Right to Die." *Insight*, October 13, 1986, 54.

Robin, Eugene D. *Medical Care Can Be Dangerous to Your Health*. (Originally published as *Matters of Life and Death*.) New York: Harper and Row, 1984.

Rosenthal, Norman E., et al. "Seasonal Affective Disorder." *Archives of General Psychiatry* 41 (January 1984): 72–79.

Rossiter, L. F.; Langwell, K.; Wan, T. T. H.; and Rivnyak, M. "Patient Satisfaction Among Elderly Enrollees and Disenrollees in Medicare Health Maintenance Organizations." *Journal of the American Medical Association* 262 (1989): 57–63.

Ruark, J.; Raffin, T.; and the Stanford University Medical Center Committee on Ethics. "Initiating and Withdrawing Life Support. Principles and Practice in Adult Medicine." *The New England Journal of Medicine* 318 (1988): 25–30.

Schiedermayer, D. "The Decision to Forgo CPR in the Elderly." *Journal of the American Medical Association* 260 (1988): 2096–97.

Schroeder, S. A.; Kenders, K.; Cooper, J. K.; et al. "Use of Laboratory

Tests and Pharmaceuticals: Variations Among Physicians and Effect of Cost Audit on Subsequent Use." *Journal of the American Medical Association* 225 (1973): 969–73.

———; Martin, K. I.; and Strom, B. L. "Frequency and Morbidity of Invasive Procedures." *Archives of Internal Medicine* 138 (1978): 1809.

Seravalli, E. P. "The Dying Patient, the Physician, and the Fear of Death." *The New England Journal of Medicine* 319 (1988): 1728–30.

Shakleton, Basil. *The Grape Cure: A Living Testament.* Wellingborough, Northamptonshire: Thorsons Publishers Ltd., 1969.

Sherer, Renslow. "Physician Use of the HIV Antibody Test." *Journal of the American Medical Association* 259 (1988): 264–65.

Siegler, Miriam, and Osmond, Humphry. *Patienthood.* New York: Macmillan, 1979.

Simeone, F. "Lumbar Disc Disease." Chap. 290 in *Neurosurgery.* Edited by R. Wilkins and S. Rengachary. New York: McGraw-Hill Book Co., 1985, 2250–59.

Sisk, T. "Knee Injuries." Chap. 56 in *Campbell's Operative Orthopaedics.* Edited by A. Crenshaw. St. Louis: C. V. Mosby Co., 1987, 2283–2496.

Skelly, F. J. "Good MD-Patient Relationship Linked to Good Outcome." *American Medical News,* June 9, 1989, 3.

Slovic, Paul; Fischoff, Baruch; and Lichtenstein, Sarah. "Facts Versus Fears: Understanding Perceived Risks." Chap. 33 in *Judgment Under Uncertainty: Heuristics and Biases.* Edited by D. Kahneman, P. Slovic, and A. Tversky. Cambridge: Cambridge University Press, 1982, 463–89.

Smith, M. J. *When I Say No, I Feel Guilty.* New York: Bantam Books, 1975.

Smith, Robert C., and Zimny, George H. "Physicians' Emotional Reactions to Patients." *Psychosomatics* 29, no. 4, (Fall 1988): 392–97.

Society for the Right to Die. *The Physician and the Hopelessly Ill Patient: Legal, Medical and Ethical Guidelines.* New York: Society for the Right to Die, 1985.

Somerville, J., ed. "News Digest: Medical Costs, Spending Rise." *American Medical News,* December 2, 1988, 2.

Taffet, G.; Teasdale, T.; and Luchi, R. "In-Hospital Cardiopulmonary Resuscitation." *Journal of the American Medical Association* 260 (1988): 2069–72.

"Telling Patients the Truth Without Destroying Their Hope." *Internal Medicine News*, August 15–31, 1989, 10.

Thomasma, D. "Beyond Medical Paternalism and Patient Autonomy: A Model of Physician Conscience for the Physician-Patient Relationship." *Annals of Internal Medicine* 98 (1983): 243–48.

Tolle, Susan W.; Elliot, Dane L.; and Hickam, David H. "Physician Attitudes and Practices at the Time of Patient Death." *Archives of Internal Medicine* 144 (December 1984): 2389–91.

Tomlinson, T., and Brody, H. "Ethics and Communication in Do-Not-Resuscitate Orders." *The New England Journal of Medicine* 318 (1988): 43–46.

Tversky, Amos, and Kahneman, Daniel. "Availability: A Heuristic for Judging Frequency and Probability." Chap. 11 in *Judgment Under Uncertainty: Heuristics and Biases.* Edited by D. Kahneman, P. Slovic, and A. Tversky. Cambridge: Cambridge University Press, 1982, 164–78.

"Understanding the Many Causes of Patient Noncompliance." *Internal Medicine News* 16, no. 9 (May 1–14, 1983): 13.

Veatch, Robert M. "Deciding Against Resuscitation: Encouraging Signs and Potential Dangers." *Journal of the American Medical Association* 253 (1985): 77–78.

———, ed. *Life Span: Values and Life-Extending Technologies.* San Francisco: Harper and Row, 1979.

VerBerkmoes, R. "Health Costs: $1.5 Trillion in Year 2000." *American Medical News*, June 19, 1987, 3.

Wanzer, S.; Adelstein, S.; Cranford, R.; et al. "The Physician's Responsibility Toward Hopelessly Ill Patients." *The New England Journal of Medicine* 310 (1984): 955–59.

———; Federman, D.; Adelstein, S.; et al. "The Physician's Responsibility Toward Hopelessly Ill Patients: A Second Look." *The New England Journal of Medicine* 320 (1989): 844–49.

Wanzer, Sidney H. "Euthanasia: The Argument in Favor." *Clinical Report on Aging* 2, no. 5 (1988): 1ff.

Weinstein, Neil. "Why It Won't Happen to Me: Perceptions of Risk Factors and Susceptibility." *Health Psychology* 3, no. 5 (1984): 431–57.

Wennberg, J.; Mulley, A.; Hanley, D.; Timothy, R.; Fowler, F.; Roos, N.; Barry, M.; McPherson, K.; Greenberg, E.; Soule, D.; Bubolz,

T.; Fisher, E.; and Malenka, D. "An Assessment of Prostatectomy for Benign Urinary Tract Obstruction. Geographic Variations and the Evaluation of Medical Care Outcomes." *Journal of the American Medical Association* 259 (1988): 3027–30.

Wennberg, John. "Dealing with Medical Practice Variations: A Proposal for Action." *Health Affairs* 3, no. 2 (Summer 1984): 6–32.

———. "Which Rate Is Right?" *The New England Journal of Medicine* 314 (1986): 310–11.

———, and Gittelsohn, A. "Small Area Variations in Health Care Delivery." *Science* 182 (1973): 1102–8.

White, William B., et al. "Daily Blood Pressure, Not Office Pressure, Determines Cardiac Function in Patients With Hypertension." *Journal of the American Medical Association* 261 (1989): 873–77.

"Will 'Right Thinking' Keep You Well?" *University of California, Berkeley, Wellness Letter,* September 1988, 1.

Winslow, C.; Kosecoff, J.; Chassin, M.; Kanouse, D.; and Brook, R. "The Appropriateness of Coronary Artery Bypass Surgery." *Journal of the American Medical Association* 260 (1988): 505–9.

Winslow, C.; Solomon, D.; Chassin, M.; et al. "The Appropriateness of Carotid Endarterectomy." *The New England Journal of Medicine* 318 (1988): 721–27.

Young, Mark J., and Poses, Roy M. "Can Physicians Be Rational About Diagnostic Tests?" *Clinics in Laboratory Medicine* 4, no. 1 (March 1984): 25–39.

Zinn, William M. "Doctors Have Feelings Too." *Journal of the American Medical Association* 259 (1988): 3296–98.

INDEX